I0500113

BARBIE & KEN—A LOVE STORY

A Couple's Journey Through Multiple Scerlosis

A True Story Told By:

Barbara Celeste McCloskey

© 2017 Barbara Celeste McCloskey
All rights reserved.

ISBN: 1548354120
ISBN 13: 9781548354121

To Ken, my love, my soul mate, my partner.
And many thanks to Marie Meyer for her love and candid support.

ENTERING THE TWILIGHT ZONE

Twelve years ago, my husband was abducted by aliens. I'm sure of it because he's never been the same since. Since that fateful day, we've forged ahead holding on to each other through each scary step.

It all started with a phone call.

"Hello, sweetheart. I need you." Ken was crying.

He never cried.

My stomach rose into my throat when I heard his voice. "Where are you?"

"I'm at the mall."

"Where at the mall?"

"I don't know. I don't even know how I got here."

He sounded like a scared five year old.

"Look around you and tell me what you see."

"I'm in the hallway outside one of the entrances, using one of the pay phones. There's a fingernail place across from me, and one of those "You Are Here" layouts in the middle of the hallway."

"Okay, that's good. Take a deep breath, and I'll be right there. Don't move."

My chest tightened as I put on my coat and flew out the door. *What in the world happened?* I jumped in my car and drove as fast as traffic allowed. My imagination operated in hyper-drive. Terrifying scenarios manifested. *Was he hurt? Had someone mugged him? Why couldn't he tell me what happened? And why didn't he know where he was?*

Five minutes later, I parked the car at the southeast entrance and ran into the building. From his description of his surroundings, I surmised he had to be somewhere close. I opened the set of glass doors and looked around. There he was sitting on a bench in the courtyard with his head down.

I walked up to him and uttered his name in a soft voice. "Ken. I'm here."

"Sweetheart!" He looked up. His eyes were watery and red. He grabbed me in a strong embrace. "I'm so glad you're here."

I looked at his troubled face. He had terror in his eyes.

"It's okay now. I'm here." He didn't let go.

I felt his body relax in our embrace. I sat on the bench and motioned for him to sit beside me. "Can you tell me anything?"

"I don't know how I got in here. I don't remember driving to the mall or where I parked the car." His voice was low and tears teetered on his eyelids. "What the hell is wrong with me?"

"What were you doing before you got to the mall?"

"Patrick and I met for coffee at Wilson's."

"Do you remember driving the car?"

He took a deep breath. "Yes."

"Do you remember the road you took to get here?"

"Yes. I drove down Green Bay Road."

As he pieced together parts of his memory, he took a deep breath.

"So you turned into the mall from the west side by Applebee's?"

"No. I turned in by Olive Garden."

"That's good. Do you remember where you parked the car?"

The tears that had been balancing on his eyelids slid down his cheeks. "I don't know!"

I put my arm around him. "It's okay. We'll find the car. Do you have a headache? Are you hurt? Perhaps I should call the ambulance and have you checked out at the hospital."

"No! No doctors. No hospital. I'm fine." He added, "Now that you're here."

Not wanting to add more distress, I took his hand and walked out of the building to my car. I could understand his angst about going to the hospital; after all, it had been a short time since he had nearly died after cancer surgery and then faced four months of chemotherapy. I opened the passenger's side of my car, and he crawled inside.

I said, "I'll just drive around and maybe you'll remember something."

He nodded.

As I circled the mall, I continued to question him to ascertain where his car might be parked. "If you came in at the other end of the mall, do you remember why you came here?"

"Yes. I wanted to buy some blades for my electric shaver."

"That's good. Do you remember which store you planned to purchase them?"

"That little store by Penny's."

"But that's on the other end of the mall from where you called me."

He began to cry again. "I can't tell you how I got on the other end of the complex. It's like I lost a chunk of time. Why is this happening?"

My voice remained calm which surprised me. "I don't know, honey. It's okay. We'll piece this thing together. Try to stay calm." I hid my concern by putting a sound of confidence in my voice. But deep down, I wondered what could have caused this fiasco.

Ken brushed away a tear rolling down his cheek. "Oh, sweetheart, I don't know what I'd do without you. I feel like I'm losing my mind."

I didn't respond. Clearly something very serious happened to him, but what? Why couldn't he remember these simple things?

We drove around the mall for about twenty minutes before we found the car. "There it is! There's the car." Ken's voice sounded like a joyous child.

"Do you remember anything more now that you see the car?"

"No."

"I don't think you should drive, Ken."

He turned and looked at me with clear eyes. "I'm fine now. I can get the car home."

"I don't know. Perhaps we should call someone to drive it home for us."

His fear turned to anger. "No. Don't treat me like a child! I can drive the damn car!" He jumped out of my car with his keys in his hand, unlocked the door to his car, and waved to me.

I followed him back to our condo and got him safely inside. When I saw him in the kitchen, he looked very weary.

"I made soup for supper. Would you like a sandwich with it?"

"No. I really don't feel like eating. I think I'll go to bed."

"Are you sure? When was the last time you had something to eat?"

"I ate my lunch at break time, like always."

"That was over seven hours ago. Why don't you go wash up, and I'll put supper on the table?"

"Maybe you're right." He hung up his jacket in the living room closet and went into the bathroom.

He ate a small bowl of soup before he went to bed. I picked up the phone and called the doctor. This unexplained event troubled me more than I could express. As an engineer, Ken was naturally meticulous with a keen attention for details. He needed to be checked out. But not tonight. He was in no danger. I would keep the vigil. Nothing or no one would harm him. Our appointment was in two days.

We never did know for sure what happened that night, but a year later he was diagnosed with a seizure disorder. We just got his seizures under control when we learned he also suffered from Multiple Sclerosis. His confusion and loss of memory could have been a result of either problem. An alien abduction would have been easier to accept because it would entail one event unlike this diagnosis which means a lifetime of degeneration. It's our walk through a personal "Twilight Zone."

THE MS BEAST

AN MS EXACERBATION. . .

I'm writing this entry after a couple of very bad days for Ken. Thankfully when he woke this morning he was feeling better, so we decided to pick-up our retired friend Joyce for a cup of coffee. We went to a quaint coffee shop, which is situated on beautiful Lake Michigan. As Ken and I walk through these hard times, Joyce supports us.

We usually sit in the backroom, so we can look out toward the lake, but today we chose to sit at an antique table in the art room. It's a peaceful room with low light. Local artists contribute to the ambiance with their exquisite paintings. Best of all Ken was in good spirits, cracking us up with his dry wit. We spent the next hour laughing together.

Unfortunately, MS decided to disrupt our visit by suddenly making Ken weak. Whenever a wave of fatigue hits him, he also has strong urge to go to the bathroom, but most of the time, it's only an urge. I helped him struggled to get to the Men's Room, but after several unsuccessful trips, I realized he was experiencing a "normal" pattern.

As the weakness got stronger, Ken couldn't walk. Luckily there were a couple of men willing to help Joyce and me get him into the car. I dropped Joyce off and headed for home. During the drive home, Ken had a pee accident, and he was humiliated. As for me, I was more worried about how I was going to get him safely into the house than I was about a wet car seat.

Ken used every ounce of the strength he had to get in the house while I pulled, pushed a supported him through the backdoor into the kitchen. After we got into the house, he collapsed on the rug in front of the kitchen sink and went to sleep. As much as I wanted to get him into bed, I needed to leave him on the floor because I couldn't lift him. His body had become a bowl of jelly, but at least he was safe, and I knew after he rested we could try again to get him up. Right now all I could do was make him comfortable with a pillow and blanket.

He woke about fifteen minutes later, and I put him on an office chair and rolled him into the bathroom to get cleaned up. Then it was back on the chair to the living room where I made him comfortable on the sofa. He was drooling and his speech was "lazy," making him hard to understand.

After a brief rest, he was able to eat a sandwich and a banana, washing the food down with a glass of milk. He still suffered from terrible urges to go to the bathroom, and he didn't want to have another accident, so I gave him his medication which helps curb the urges. He still fought me to walk to the bathroom. Did I mention my husband can be very stubborn?

Finally, I lost it. I yelled at him. I was scared and exhausted, but as soon as the words were out of my mouth, I felt ashamed for blowing my top, but my outburst kept him stay on the sofa and he consented to using the plastic urinal. After he relaxed, he finally succumbed to taking a nap with the hope he'd feel stronger once he woke.

I watched him sleep for about ninety minutes, and when he woke, he still couldn't walk, but he could talk in a tone and intonation I could understand.

"I'm sorry sweetheart" were the first words out of his mouth.

"I am, too, Ken." I walked over and kissed him.

"I'm such a load. It shouldn't be like this for you."

"It shouldn't be like this for you, either, but we did promised "for better or for worse," didn't we?"

He smiled. "I guess we did."

"Tomorrow will be better."

"Yeah. Tomorrow will be better."

We both sighed and our dilemma was over for today.

A DIFFERENT KIND OF ROADSTER

I've been exploring the possibility of acquiring a handicapped van, so Ken and I can get out and enjoy some of the things we love to do together. He spends a good time in his power wheelchair now, and needless to say it doesn't fit in our little Mitsubishi. When we go out, the trip ends up to be a trial for both of us. Either I need to hoist a manual wheel chair into the car and push it around, or he must struggle with his walker.

Come to find out, there is a used car lot in Racine which handles such vehicles. I found a van yesterday, but it was thirteen years old, and it had a funny smell. I walked away because I'm not ready to give up my SUV. The other part of my decision was I'm not comfortable realizing we truly need such equipment sooner than later. This is another instance which shines a light on the fact Ken's MS is progressing.

One thing is for sure, this MS journey has taught me to wait. I have confidence the time will come when everything seems right, and I'll be able to make the right decision for us. Until that day comes, we'll struggle along with what we have and be thankful.

CONSTANT CHANGE

During our years together, Ken and I have divided the household chores. I do the cooking, and he does the dishes. I do the dusting, he cleans the bathroom. I do the vacuuming, and he does the laundry. But as Ken's MS progresses, going down to the basement to do the laundry has become perilous. His balance is impaired, and I'm afraid he may take a tumble.

As soon as we can, we plan to bring our washer and dryer upstairs, so he can feel productive again. We've had an assessment completed by the state, and the representative agreed it is important for Ken to contribute to our relationship by doing the household chores he can do. Therefore, they agreed to pay for the "infrastructure" work—plumbing and electrical changes, but we would have to buy the machines. We can do that. I still have a little money in my retirement account.

We found a contractor we like, so our project starts in another month. In the meantime, Ken and I search the newspaper ads and various appliance store websites for a good deal on new machines.

I think we're having almost as much fun planning the remodeling project as we will be using the new space.

It's fun to still dream and plan together. Doing so has always been one of the things we enjoy, and I'm so grateful MS hasn't taken that away from us.

A SHADE OF GRAY ON A SUNNY DAY

As I reflect on the pieces I've included in this book, I realize I talk a lot about the weather. I hope you don't mind. Whether it's sunny and warm, gray and rainy, or frigidly cold, weather affects my mood.

Take yesterday. We were blessed with a bright sunny day after suffering several days of gray days. Ken and I hadn't been out of the house for many days in a row, so we decided it would be nice to go out for lunch and run a couple of errands. Unfortunately, the way it turned out, we should have stayed home.

We didn't argue; don't get that idea. But by the time we got to the restaurant, Ken suffered a wave of fatigue. We both attributed his weariness to being hungry, but it turned out to be more than that.

Multiple Sclerosis spoiled the day--again. Ken actually fought to keep his eyes open while we sat at the table. We both looked so forward to being out of the house, and now this damn disease unexpectedly captured my husband and took him away from me. Today turned out to be a day when Ken needed me to feed him.

He was embarrassed, and I was frustrated on the inside. Luckily, my vocal chords took a day off, and we finished our lunch not talking to each other. I helped him to the car, drove home, and put him to bed. I wanted to cry, but I've learned not to waste the energy because I know such disappointments will come again.

Some people tell me I should write our experience because through my words, I have the power to help others. That might be true, if it weren't so painful, Writing about disappointments is difficult. I hate admitting my failings and standing by as I watch my dear husband slip away.

To write the true story I need to include the good times and the bad. If I didn't, I'd let other caretakers down. If I can offer comfort or inspire with one entry in this book, I have done my job.

Honestly, though, events like today make me want to feel like this is a bad idea.

ARE WE REALLY "RETIRED"?

This morning we started our day by heading out to the hospital for Ken to have an EEG. The orders were for him to have no caffeine for eight hours, limit sleep to four hours, and show up with clean hair. He did very well — but me? Well, I've gotten real good at "sleeping in" until eight o'clock, so I was pretty groggy. I made my way to the garage like a zombie, loaded his wheelchair on the lift, and we were on our way at 6:30 a.m.

When I worked outside our home, I was up, showered, dressed, and eating breakfast at this hour. But since I've been home with Ken, we've gotten very comfortable in our slow "retirement" life. Even though I'm employed by the state for Ken's care, I consider myself retired. My time is my own; I don't have to answer to a boss; and best of all I don't have to commute for an hour one way. I'll admit I've become pretty soft.

I never received a retirement party or gold watch and my employment ended before I was ready, but I couldn't buy a job in 2009. Deep down I assured myself my unemployment was God's way of telling me I was needed more at home than on any other position.

The experience has been good for me, though. My blood pressure is down and I have learned to keep myself content. Best of all, I get to be with Ken. People often ask me if I resent not getting to live out a more "traditional" retirement. My come back is: "What is a traditional retirement?" They often mention travel and volunteering. Of course, Ken and I wish we could live out our dreams of traveling, but we did a lot of it before he got so sick. We missed an Alaska excursion and a river cruise in Europe, but that's okay. We travel via the Travel Channel and Aerial America on television. Sure, we'd like to go to the places we visit via digital images, but we're content to live within our changing parameters.

After his test, we treated each other to breakfast at our favorite eatery and then enjoyed the afternoon with a nap. A good day.

SEEING A CRASH – LAUGH

Today, I woke to the thud—again. Multiple Sclerosis has made this a common sound in our household, but to wake to a crash is worse than any alarm clock. The sound reminds me of the "sonic booms" I heard as a child when faster-than-the-speed-of-sound jets used to fly over our house. The windows would rattle and no matter what you were doing at the time, you stopped for a few seconds to make sure the sky wasn't falling. Ken's falls are like that for me.

One of my favorite movies is called "*Cool Runnings*." It's a Disney film about the Jamaican bobsled team. They trained for the Olympic Games with a rickety "push cart" they piloted in local competitions. This push cart was basically a few wooden crates with four wheels and a steering mechanism. They propelled the contraption down winding hills, often crashing. After they came to a jarring stop, one of the fellows says to another, "Maurice, are you dead?" The answer is always, "Ya, mon." It cracks me up every time.

So now when Ken crashes, I yell, "Kenneth, are you dead?"

This morning he played along and said, "Ya, mon!"
We both laughed hard and loud, checking nothing was damaged but his pride and went to the kitchen for breakfast.
    Laughter saves us every time.

WATCHING HIM SLIP AWAY

Most of the time I go from day to day without thinking about the things I need to do for Ken now which I didn't do a year ago. The latest challenge is he often finds it hard to swallow. Such losses make me realize he will continue to fail until I can't be the person who cares for him any longer.

Death of a loved one is difficult to accept in any situation, but I think watching the degenerative progression of disease in someone you love is worse. It's like I lose him a bit each day.

Ken always loved doing little things for me--like buying a corsage for me the first time he heard me sing a solo. Like buying me a dress I loved but didn't need; in fact he ran around with the dress in the trunk of his car until he could give it to me on my birthday. He took the effort to know me well enough to ALWAYS give me something I loved—whether it was a hug, a smile, or a little remembrance. I miss his thoughtfulness. I miss my husband.

I know as time goes on everyone will experience caretaking on some level--either as the recipient or the one giving the care. Not being independent enough to do simple things like cutting meat at dinner or putting on his own shoes every day is humiliating. Ken never talks about these occurrences, and I can't imagine how he truly feels because he never complains.

If Ken were a different person, I don't think I could do all that is required. He is the sweetest most loving man I've ever met. I loved him when we married almost twenty years ago, and through the years our love has grown exponentially. Our love keeps me steady. I'm no hero. I'm no saint. I just love the man I married. That's all.

HUNKERIN' DOWN

This summer didn't show up until a few weeks ago. Our temperatures were in the high 60s and low 70s, which is perfect in my book. But since Thursday, things have changed. We Wisconsinites are not used to temperatures in the 90s for any length of time and this week the mercury soared into that stratosphere.

Usually when temperatures get this hot, we have a big thunderstorm, and it cools off. Not this time. Oh, we did get a thunderstorm bad enough to haul out our dog Ernie's "thunder jacket," but instead of cooling off, the temperature returned to its high intensity. MS patients don't do well in the heat, so Ken and I are marooned in the air conditioning until the weather gets more like Wisconsin instead of Florida.

Luckily, we don't have a problem keeping busy because we both have our own distractions. I'm still reeling from the flu so I don't have to feel guilty by spending another day on the sofa. Ken spends the day on his computer, and Ernie only needs to go outside a couple of times in between naps. So it'll be another quiet day.

I can live with that.

HOSTING A PARTY

Ken comes from a very closely knit family. Everybody enjoys being together. There's no "in" fighting or back biting. We love to play together. I've been privileged to be part of such a group for over twenty years.

We always celebrate birthdays during the season they occur. Summer birthdays usually in July, Fall birthdays in September, etc. This summer I wanted to host the get together because I can handle a crowd with our big backyard and our new "Taj Garage." So we hosted a picnic for all the Cancers and Leos in the family.

Today we were supposed to go down to Steve and Tara's home. (Steve is Ken's brother.) We planned to celebrate the Autumn birthdays. Ken was moving extremely slow, but he was in good spirits, and he really wanted to make the trip, so I consented and asked my friend Jackie to make the trip with us. Driving almost hundred miles one way is a little much for me these days. Fighting Chicago traffic makes the top ten things I least want to do.

I put his power wheelchair in the car and watched him move toward the front seat. I didn't know he was hanging onto the back door, and I pushed the button to automatically open it for him to put in the walker. And wham! He screamed at me for opening the door which caused him to lose his balance. I gasped as he fell and his head bounced on the concrete floor. Ken just accomplished one of my biggest fears – hitting his head on something when he falls.

I became frantic digging out my cellphone from my purse and dialed 911. In minutes the rescue squad came and checked him out. A quick swelling lump and a bit of blood freaked me out. The good news was — it was only a bump. No concussion. The paramedics handed him an ice pack and got him safely into the house. And do you believe it? He still wanted to make the trip.

I yelled, "No!" I still shook from fear. "We're staying home. Neither of us are in any shape to go to a party."

The trip would have been good for us, but I was traumatized. The whole experience took the wind out of my sails. My "fight or flight" instinct kicked in. I wanted to run away. Even though I knew this urge would pass, I allowed myself to feel it. I can't sweep my fears under the carpet because there's already a big lump of unresolved feelings under there already.

We each took a deep breath and calmed down as the afternoon wore on. We ate lunch and settled into our recliners to watch a movie. Hours passed. By sundown we got to a normal place, kissed each other, and went to bed dreaming of a better day tomorrow.

HEAT AND MS DON'T MIX

This September day is one of nature's last hurrahs as the temperature climbed into the high 80s. Unfortunately, the warmth means Ken needs to remain in the house in the air conditioning. For most MS patients heat is lethal. It brings on paralyzing fatigue, and Ken succumbs to such weather.

His sister called on Saturday, saying she and her family, along with Ken's parents wanted to visit on Sunday. We grew excited as we waited for their visit. Sue suggested we go out for lunch, but I knew Ken's reaction to the summer temperatures wouldn't be favorable, so I suggested I make lunch, and they bring dessert.

Unfortunately I was right about Ken's reaction to the heat. He woke suffering from a terrible bought of fatigue. It wasn't the worst case he ever had, but from the time he woke to the time he went to bed, he fought to keep his eyes open. I made him lie down after breakfast with the hope he might fall asleep for a little while, but he couldn't sleep. You see "fatigue" is very different than being tired. Fatigue doesn't mean you're sleepy; it means every move becomes difficult–even keeping one's eyes open is hard. Even forming words and speaking can be difficult. In a word fatigue SUCKS.

By the time the family arrived, Ken mustered enough strength to enjoy the visit. Like always, he found strength and happiness having his family close. When they left around five in the afternoon, Ken relaxed in his chair. We watched numbing reruns on television, and he didn't fight the battle of fatigue any longer. We went to bed at eight o'clock, and as soon as his head hit the pillow, he fell asleep.

I stayed awake and held his hand. I file away all moments like this one. Darkness in the quiet night makes everything all right. The solace I find there makes a perfect end to a challenging day.

MS – A SOB

Did you ever have a day when you just wanted to run away from your life? Yeah. Me, too. In fact, today is one of those days.

I woke up this morning before six o'clock to the sound of Ken struggling. I rushed to the kitchen and saw him hanging onto the counter. In seconds he was destined to hit the tile. I think I lose a part of my life every time he tumbles, so I pulled over one of the kitchen chairs with casters to catch him.

One slight little turn or wobble and down he goes. Luckily, most of his falls leave him unscathed. I think he has a legion of guardian angels on the job to break his falls. Today I stood in for those angels who often must work overtime to keep him safe.

Ken managed to make coffee and put his breakfast dishes on the table, but he hadn't eaten yet. On top of that, the dog was dancing to go outside and the cat was meowing for his morning tuna. For some reason, today these normal occurrences were too much for me. I barely had my eyes open and my morning already spun out of control through no fault of my own.

I think MS stands for Mean Son-of-a-Bitch because that is exactly what a patient and his family around him/her experience.

Yelling is a release, but it does little good. Huffing and puffing doesn't help either. Nothing helps when you find yourself in a whirling moment. I'm no saint. I lose it once in a while.

Taking deep breaths helps. A couple cups of coffee helps. But it's usually a dash of quiet time that helps me put things in perspective. When I have found that nice person inside me who I like a lot better than the crazy woman who took over this morning, I can smile and be pleasant.

I still would dream about a vacation, though — perhaps a nice sail down a lazy river? Yeah. I'll meditate on that.

OIL CHANGES AND OTHER ADVENTURES

Since Ken's fall last Sunday, I've been a space cadet. I knew I was upset when he went down in the garage and his noggin hit the pavement, but I never dreamed I'd become stupid.

Let me share a story.

Because car repairs now end up in my "in box," it was time for an oil change and a tire rotation. I received a coupon which would save me forty bucks if I made it into the dealership before the end of September. I called my friend Pam to pick me up after I dropped off the car, so we could have a cup of coffee while the car waited its turn to have the transfusion and tire adjustment.

We both took off from my house and traveled west. I pulled into the driveway of the garage and thought, "This doesn't look right. Oh well, I haven't been out here for quite a while, maybe they did some renovations to the building." I drove through the unfamiliar entrance and got out of the car to talk to the intake manager. It went like this:

"Good afternoon, Miss." (I love it when they don't call me "ma'am.") "What can we do for you today?"

I answered. "I have a 2:30 appointment for an oil change and tire rotation."

"Name?"

"Barbara McCloskey."

"How do you spell that?"

"M C C L O S K E Y."

He rattled a few keys on the computer and his face went blank. "You're not in the computer."

Nothing's worse than being absent in the all-knowing computer. "I don't understand. I called yesterday and talked to Patty."

"We don't have a Patty on staff."

Now I really thought I lost my mind. "I don't understand. I talked at Patty at Palmen Service Department and signed up to bring my car in at 2:30."

He still wore a blank expression. "Palmen?"

"Yes."

"Ma'am. (Oh god, now I'm ma'am.) You're at Boucher. Palmen is two blocks that way." He pointed east.

Without thinking I said, "Well that explains everything, doesn't it?" I actually didn't blush. "I'm at the wrong dealership. Chalk it up to a senior moment."

I got in my car and exited the service bay. In my rear view mirror, I saw the service manager laughing as he talked to one of his colleagues. Great! Now I won the reputation of a crazy lady.

A few minutes later I pulled into the right dealership. Honked the horn to get them to open the door. Drove in. Got out and repeated the process.

The guy says, "Your name is in not in the computer."

"I talked to Patty yesterday and made the appointment."

"We have two Patties."

"Good. I talked to one of them."

"Hmmmm." The guy tapped on the computer a bit. "We can fit you in."

"I have a coupon for the oil change and tire rotation."

"All right."

I dug in my purse. Ken calls my purse the black hole, and today he was right. I had no coupon. Then I remembered I left it on my desk. "When I come back, I'll bring the coupon."

He must have sensed I was having a bad day. "That will be fine, ma'am."

I smiled and called Pam because she was nowhere to be seen. "Hi, my friend. Where are you?"

"The question is where *are you*?"

"I'm at Palmen where I'm supposed to be."

"I saw you drive into Boucher and then I lost you."

"Just come to Palmen, and I'll wait outside for you."

"Okay." She hung up.

Two seconds later, we made contact. I opened the passenger's door and plopped down in the seat. "I need a drink. Not coffee."

THE BEAUTY AND THE BEAST

Autumn is my favorite time of the year. Temperatures cool and landscapes put on brilliant colors. It's a time when Ken and I love to go for a car ride. The gold, red, and orange leaves paint the hills and entertain us for hours. Today was a good day for a ride. As we meandered through the country roads, I wondered how many people just drive by the trees and never give the surrounding beauty a thought. Needless to say, drivers who were behind me weren't looking at the leaves. One driver passed me with his middle finger raised defiantly.

We invited my "big sister" Joyce to come along with us. She doesn't drive any longer because a nasty stroke took away some of her vision in one eye. We've enjoyed this outing together for the past few years, so now it's become a tradition. We ooooo'd and ahhhh'd over nature's handiwork and then treated ourselves to a cup of coffee afterward.

The outing was a success until we arrived back at Joyce's house. Ken had to use the bathroom, but because he wasn't having the best of days, he didn't make it inside the house. Consequently, we took a rain check on the coffee and went home.

I know these accidents aren't his fault, but they often are a source of frustration. I hated to have to cut our outing short. I hated feeling this way, but it seems I turn invisible as the caretaker.

The only reason I bring up this subject is because I know other caretakers feel this way too — only few of us express how we really feel. We swallow the disappointments (and there are many) and one day we have to admit we can't assume the role anymore. No matter how much one person loves another there are limits.

This afternoon I found one of my limits. Nobody can fix this situation and give me my REAL husband back. Disease doesn't work that way. It just keeps rolling along until it runs you over. Unlike rude drivers, this vehicle doesn't care who's in the way.

A DAY AT A TIME

The title of this piece has become a cliché in our world, but when tough times come along it truly is the best way to live.

The intent of this book is to share our experience with MS trying to maintain an upbeat perspective, but if I only talk about the good times, this book wouldn't be a truthful account. Let's face it; sometimes life drops a load of crap on us no matter if we are rich or poor, sick or healthy, positive or negative. There are times of indecision, confusion, and frustration. Nobody wants to admit weakness and failure, but it happens. In other words, dealing with MS is a tough experience.

The biggest challenge is never knowing what kind of day we're going to get. Yesterday Ken woke feeling well, but as the morning went on, a crushing wave of fatigue washed over him, and his day changed drastically. It happens. Often. Unless a person witnesses this transformation up close and personal, you might not believe it truly happens.

During the bad times, we pull together and hang on. He stays safe in his wheelchair, and I do everything I can to keep him comfortable.

There are millions of people caring for someone they love. I can only speak from my perspective, so I can share what important lessons I've learned. Maybe our story might help you. Here are a few lessons we've learned the hard way.

- We've learned to live in the present.
- We've learned we need others to help us.
- We've learned to keep positive even in tough times.
- We've learned how to work with professional people to get what we need to keep going.

Here's what I've learned being a caretaker.

- I must be good to myself.
- I need time away to maintain a positive attitude.
- I shouldn't beat up myself for losing my temper. When I lose it, I apologize and try to forgive myself.
- Small accomplishments should never be minimized.

Remember a strong relationship takes two partners willing to work with each other. A healthy union means giving and taking. Finding contentment in the mundane is necessary. And above all else, we have learned to take one day at a time. The phrase has become trite, but it is not. It's a survival tactic.

BECOMING HUMBLE

"God opposes the proud but gives grace to the humble."
(James 4:6).

Ordinarily, I don't quote the bible because I think it's pretentious to do so. Growing up Catholic I was taught reading the bible was only for "trained personnel" like priests and nuns. But today, when I saw this quote, I had to pass it on because it fits what I've been experiencing this week.

We've had to accept help from energy assistance to keep warm, food stamps to put gifts on our dining table, and prescription help to keep Ken functioning. The last few years have humbled me. Now the only thing pride does is get in my way to keep us going.

Every time I need to reach out for help, a big lump in my throat makes me feel like I can't swallow. I'm ashamed I'm not as strong as I thought I was. I don't even know enough to navigate out of this place we're in.

The grace we receive comes through our true friends. They have proven they are a well-equipped army standing beside us, springing into action the second we need them. They hold us up when we can't stand on our own any longer. Their generosity over-whelms us, and the words, "Thank You" hardly seem adequate. Best of all, they help us see there is light at the end of the tunnel, and it isn't another train coming to mow us down.

Going through the MS experience without our friends and Ken's loving family would indeed be a nightmare.

JOY TURNED TO MISERY

After breakfast, I got dressed and planted the perennials I purchased yesterday. The shaded backyard was just the right temperature and planting flowers always makes me happy. I kept thinking about next year when these posies would be in full bloom.

When I returned to the house, I found Ken dressed and sitting on the bedroom floor.

"What happened to you, dear?"

"I missed the vanity chair and landed on my butt. I can't seem to get myself up."

Yes. It was time to call 911 again and ask for another "lift assist."

After the rescue team left, Ken drove his wheelchair out to the living room. He looked exhausted, and began speaking with a "thick tongue." Instantly, I knew we were in for a long day, especially when he didn't argue with me to take a time out and rest on the sofa.

An hour later, he attempted to get up and couldn't. He wedged his body between his chair and the sofa while attempting to make a trip to the bathroom. Needless to say, he didn't make it and now we had another problem.

As I tried to strip him down, wash him, and then put on clean disposable underwear and slacks, he was like a 170 lb. ball of jelly. He couldn't move his body, but after a few attempts and deep breaths, I did manage to get him changed and comfortable again.

He said he was hungry, but it took him about a half an hour to eat half a sandwich. He returned to the sofa and remained in this stupor for several hours. He even thought I was his Mom. He kept asking for Barb — and there I was right in front of him. I wanted to cry. Not only was his body malfunctioning, his mind was playing tricks on him, too.

All I can say is, I hope we don't have one of these days again for a long, long time. It's too heartbreaking.

NEVER MINIMIZE GOOD TIMES

Ken has had a good week. He hasn't fallen once. This is a gift. Believe me. Every time he falls, my heart skips a beat.

We went out for lunch yesterday, but I can see our outing has taken a toll. He's struggling to charge his power wheelchair and then walk four feet to his recliner. If he does complain, which is hardly ever, he says he feels "off." Can you imagine that? I can't. He is such minimalist.

As time goes on, he's losing the ability to walk at all. It's like his feet and his brain are on two different frequencies and needless to say, his thoughts and actions don't communicate.

Now he can't stand up and give me a hug and kiss because his balance is so poor. Sometimes his speech is slurred, and I can't understand him. When I tell him so, he must focus to get the words out. But at least these episodes aren't too frequent. I don't think either of us could tolerate that.

But the times when debilitating fatigue takes over are the worst. I fear someday these symptoms will become the norm. I fear someday he'll have to go to a nursing home because I can't take care of him anymore. I'm hoping by that time, we can afford to have the necessary equipment moved in along with a 24-hour nurse.

I think uncertainty is the real culprit of my angst. I've found when I understand a situation, I find ways to cope. But this enemy is tricky. A symptom might appear today and scare the heck out of us, only to vanish the next day. One symptom we've encountered a couple of times is uncontrollable crying. It's called PBA. We got medication for it, but later found out the psych drugs he must take which help him focus and speak rationally are not compatible with the PBA drug. So we stopped it. Luckily, Ken hasn't suffered the disturbing crying episode again.

We work at keeping normalcy, even though our situation is anything but normal. And you know, most of the time it works. When it doesn't, we look forward to a better day tomorrow.

PENNIES FROM HEAVEN

Believe it or not, seven hundred dollars land in my lap. Here's what happened. Ken and I bought a wheelchair van. (That story appears in a later piece in the book.)

A couple of days after the purchase, I studied the papers I had signed with unemotional eyes and found a mistake; they only gave me six thousand for the trade-in, so I called the salesman right away and told him of the discrepancy. Because I discovered the mistake in the middle of Labor Day weekend, I would have to wait until the following Tuesday to get the problem rectified.

The following Tuesday I got my good self out to the dealership. The salesman met me at my car with a big smile and said, "Barb, you were exactly right. The loan guy found the mistake, and you'll get a check in a couple of days." We shook on it, and I went home.

As you might imagine, seven hundred dollars is a lot of money for me, so I waited for the postman everyday like a lovesick teen-ager waiting for a letter from her boyfriend. When two weeks went by and no check appeared, I called the General Manager and told him my story. While I waited on the phone, the manager confirmed the details with the salesman and said "There would be a check waiting for you at the cashier's office the next morning. You have my apologies for the delay."

"Thank you so much." I replied, hung up, and yelled, "Yippee!" Bright and early, around nine o'clock, I pointed the van west and was off to the pick up the check. I immediately plopped it in the bank and now my savings account is fatter than it has been in over five years.

As I was doing the dance of joy over that feat, Tom from Erickson Mobility came to our house to see whether he could fix Ken's power wheelchair to fit into the van. He almost had to take the whole chair apart, but he found a way to lower the seat a couple of notches, so now the magic chariot could be lifted into the van on the lift. Not only did Tom fix the chair, he adjusted the lift and told us the car might be older, but the lift was only two years old–and get this, he remembered installing it. Yippee–again!

Well, Ken and I couldn't let these two wonderful events go by without celebrating, so we got dolled up and went out for an inaugural date. We decided on having a light supper at IHOP because I had a BOGO (buy one get one) coupon. If we had been at a five-star restaurant, we wouldn't have been any happier. I love it when good things fall into my lap, don't you?

CHERISH SMALL EVENTS

I've never thought of myself as a patient person, but nowadays I take a deep breaths many times per day as I wait for Ken to complete the simplest things – like getting dressed, going to the bathroom, or taking a shower—I want to charge in and do these things for him. But I can't. Most of us take these daily occurrences for granted, but Ken has to concentrate *haaaaard* on each little step of the process to maintain some sense of independence.

I've learned to restrain myself and stand by, only responding when he asks for help. Human dignity requires all of us to have a purpose, and Ken's purpose is to be as independent as possible. So, I hold my breath as he stumbles and pray he doesn't fall.

Ken is extraordinary. He never whines or complains. He rarely voices his frustrations as MS steals more of his natural abilities away. He's my hero. I marvel at the way he lives his life happily without abilities he used to have. I don't think I would have such courage if our roles were reversed.

We can all learn from Ken. Finding success in small accomplish-ments is something most of us brush aside, but I have learned "purpose" leads the way to confidence, fulfillment, and contentment.

GOALS, PLANS, EXPECTATIONS, OH MY!

I think we humans are a curious lot. When the snow is falling, we're perusing seed catalogs for our spring gardens. When it's sweltering hot in the summer, we're purchasing snow blowers. We buy flannel pajamas in spring and swimming suits in winter. Prepare, prepare, prepare. Control, control, control. Yikes! Does anybody else think this is just a little bit crazy?

What I'm talking about it letting go of trying to control every-thing. Being in a caregiving partnership with Ken, requires us to be tolerant and flexible. "Hiccups" often upset our plans, so we do our best to adapt and roll with the change. Having a Plan "B" is a good idea when Plan "A" isn't available.

What do I mean? Well, if we are planning to meet his family for a special occasion, in case we can't go I make a point of having the ingredients for a special meal on hand. If we planned to go to a movie with friends and Ken feels too weak to go out, we invite them over and rent a movie "on demand" with our cable service.

Instead of traveling long distances, we watch "Aerial America" on television.

Learning to look down the road instead of concentrating on the hood ornament takes practice, but it is a valuable skill to acquire. No matter where the journey of life takes a person, eventually there will be a detour.

TRY NOT TO RUN

Before I crawl out of the warm blankets and put my big toe on the cold hardwood floor every morning, I let the silence of the morning wash over me. I let my brain wake up slowly with the rest of me to enjoy the sheer luxury of a soft bed, warm fleece blankets, and our little pug Ernie snoring softly by my side.

Let's face it, we all have periods when life rains down on us, and we have to make a choice. Do we lie down and quit? Or, do we get up and find a creative way to crawl out of the pit?

We've experienced many instances which have made it quite clear we're dealing with a mean, progressive disease which has brought uncertainty, unemployment, and poverty. Ken's health spirals down a bit each day, but somehow he accepts his situation. He's not selfish like I am. I wish I had a magic wand or a fairy godmother to change our situation.

I long for the kind of retirement we planned. We wanted to travel. We wanted enough money so we didn't have to pinch pennies. We always knew we were compatible to spend our days together, but we never dreamed we'd have to share our "golden years" dealing with never-ending handicaps.

MS has been an educator. It has ferreted out our true friends. When illness strikes, some friends get stupid because they don't know what to say or do, so they run away. We realized we are blessed with a stable of steady, good friends who are strong enough to walk this journey with us. We also have an extended family who chooses to love us unconditionally. Without them, our situation would be much more difficult.

So we stay the course and do our best. So far, so good, knowing someday will bring even more challenging situations.

A DEFINITION

Today I had a telephone conversation with a representative from my publisher. During our discussion, I told her I was Ken's caretaker and had started a book about our experience with this disease. She confessed she didn't know what MS really is.

I found myself giving her a primer on the disease. I'll share what I told her in case you don't understand the ins and outs of MS. Multiple Sclerosis results when lesions form in the brain or spinal column, the connections stop working normally. The myelin coating on the nerves wears away. A good visual would be an electrical cord with cracks and breaks in the plastic which coats the wire. With such damage, the cord cannot conduct electricity properly. Sometimes it works, more often it doesn't.

The disease is very hard to diagnose because the symptoms patients display are not alike. If a lesion forms in the brain, the person's cognitive ability may be impaired. If it forms around the optic nerve, the patient can go blind. If a lesion forms on the spinal cord, a patient might not be able to walk. Why people get MS is a mystery. There are new drugs to slow the disease down, but no cure.

After I finished this explanation, there was silence on the other end of the phone. The representative finally said, "I never knew that."

I smiled and said, "Glad I could help. Have a good day."

I didn't tell her this book is by far the hardest thing I've ever attempted to write.

THE BEAST OF DISEASE

Writing about my husband's struggle with Multiple Sclerosis takes the wind out of my sails. Ken keeps a positive outlook, but I need to work at it, especially on days like today. After I woke, I found him lying on the kitchen floor too weak to get up. The MS varmint bit him again and proclaimed, "I do exist!"

Every day Ken deals his balance issues, tremors in his arms, memory and cognitive issues, and most recently weakness in his legs. Once in a while the tremors are so bad he needs me to feed him. And through all of it, he never complains. I watch in wonder as he carries on. I don't know how he does it.

His upbeat attitude and his ability to laugh at himself, helps both of us. People believe I'm the strong one, but in reality it's Ken who's the rock. I gain my strength from him, and so far, we've muddled through this horrible adventure together. When a new disability appears, we creatively compensate for it. I over protect him, and he protests that I do. We blaze the trail together with supportive friends and loving relatives.

We've adjusted to a simple home life. We make a party out of planning dinners or watching Sunday football games with friends.

We rent movies and watch them on our large television screen. We laugh at the antics of our dog and cat. We find joy in a game of Scrabble. We're together and that's what really matters.

I don't think this disease is a life lesson; instead, it's a human frailty. We don't ask, "Why us?" I don't think either of us was chosen to inspire others. So far, I haven't found a message is this heartbreak. I have no advice to give. The best thing I can do is write our story. What is the same is the emotional roller coaster we all ride. It climbs and plunges, and we can't anticipate the next peak or valley. The experience is wild and scary, and the only thing we can do is hold on.

FREE FALLING

Today Ken fell five times. Every time he hit the floor, my heart stopped. Surprising, he says he feels good today. It doesn't make sense. If he feels well, why does he fall?

I think he really doesn't recognize the precarious positions he puts himself in. By the time he calls for help, he's tried so long to get up he's exhausted. He weighs one hundred seventy pounds, and I can't lift him. The best I can do is coach him how to get in the best position, so he can get up himself. Or I must call 911 for help.

The first time I called the rescue service, the men came in a ladder truck as long as our city lot is wide. Four burly guys walked up the ramp, came into the house, and in two minutes they had Ken in his chair.

The experience leaves us both spent. I never cry, but I want to. I want all of this sadness, frustration, and weakness to leave both of us. But it won't go away. We're stuck in MS quicksand. I save my tears for sappy, sentimental commercials and poignant movie scenes. That's when I shed all those tears I've stored up from days like today. This works for me. Nobody is the wiser, and I rid myself of the load I volunteered to carry.

BLAZING A
NEW TRAIL

PREMONITIONS ARE A NUDGE FROM A HIGHER POWER

Ken and I were enjoying a hamburger at a fast food restaurant when a nagging feeling interruped my thoughts. Finally I said, "Do you feel well enough to go to Palmen Motors to look at the vans on the lot? I just want to see what they have."

He answered "Sure."

And we were on our way. We were greeted by an older salesman who had a kind face. "What can I do for you tonight?"

I said. "I'm looking for a used van which I can turn into a wheelchair van."

The man's mouth dropped open. "I don't believe this! One of those came in today. We might get one per year, and this one is in terrific condition!"

I smiled. "Let's talk."

The salesman told me we could test drive the car tomorrow. On the way home Ken asked, "You knew didn't you?"

I smiled. "Know what?"

"About the car. You knew they had a van for us."

"I've learned never to dismiss my intuition. I believe God is whispering in my ear."

"Well, whatever it is, this time it really paid off."

"Don't get too excited. We haven't seen the car yet. After all, the salesman said it is quite old."

We both laughed with our fingers crossed.

When we saw the van the next day, we couldn't believe how lucky we were. Even though the car was thirteen years old, it only had 54,000 miles on it and the interior looked like it was never driven. The Chrysler Town and Country looked brand new inside. We wanted it so much!

We returned to the dealership and the quest to make this car ours began. I was upfront about our financial problems, and he said, "I promise, we'll get you and your husband into that van." Our financial department can work magic."

A manager assessed the Outlander and gave us sixty-seven hundred for it. (This was two thousand more than a previous assessment of our car at a different dealership.) Their financial manager worked hard to find us a loan at 11.9%; I anticipated we'd have to pay over twenty percent because of our recent terrible credit history. The payment came to a hundred dollars a month. I was so thrilled I could make this deal, I signed the financial papers before they could change their minds!

Long story short—the salesman made good on his promise and that evening we drove out of the dealership with a vehicle which will help us get around for years to come.

Never dismiss your intuition.

THE ROADS LESS TRAVELED

The diagnosis of MS really doesn't mean anything when you first hear the words leave the doctor's mouth. As I've said, it is a confusing and frustrating disease. Slowly this weird neurological disease quietly steals my husband away from me a bit at a time. MS is a cruel, scary enemy.

I found out I do have patience, but it only stretches so far. I have faced years slipping into poverty—a land I never inhabited before. It pains me not to have the money we need. Why must people get sucked into a "poverty black hole" simply because someone in the family got sick or injured? I don't think being sick should come with a first class ticket to the world of poverty, but it does.

Our destiny is to travel the many roads in front of us, making decisions which seem appropriate at the time. We both would rather not take this trip, but life had other ideas for us.

TEAMWORK

One of my chores today is making a "drug run" for Ken's medication. Our caring psychiatrist gives us samples because we can't afford the costly drugs which keep Ken functioning. You see, MS can manifest itself into perplexing symptoms of confusion, depression, focusing problems, and racing thoughts. The drugs he takes are not only expensive; they are extremely potent.

While I'm away, Ken plans to do a few things around the house. We're still a team. He empties the dishwasher, so later I will load it. He cleans the cat litter—please understand he volunteered for this duty—and I keep the food bowls and water full. He sorts and washes the laundry, and I help fold it. I cook and clean up. Ken and I never keep score as to who's doing what; we just do what we can at the time, and the other person picks up the slack. It's a happy situation which has worked well for almost twenty years.

As I watch Ken wither away from day to day, I marvel at his determination and strength to hold up his end of our marriage agreement. He's my every day hero, and I tell him so often. What I never tell him is my worst fear, and that's when the McCloskey team will consist of only one.

THE GOOD, THE BAD,
AND THE FRUSTRATING

A friend of mine encouraged me to write this book. She said my personal experience with caregiving might help others in the same situation. But, this book has proven to be tougher than I ever thought it would be. Writing about myself and Ken's challenges can be triumphant, but most of the time our experience is mundane. We're just living the life God put in our path. It's also hard to write about the times when things don't go smoothly. But if my friend is right and this book can help someone else who must walk this precarious journey with someone they love, the pain and effort will be worth it.

Once I got going, I realize putting down our day-to-day events is cathartic for me. But balance is essential. I don't want to sugarcoat the good times or exaggerate the frustrating and fearful times. I also want to help other caregivers understand their feelings are "normal." And that includes the days when I want to run away and never look back. It also includes those horrendous days when I might yell at Ken for making yet another mess that will cost money to get things fixed. I know when I get that low, I allow myself some distance to take a deep breath and remember I'm only human. Afterward, I go and apologize for losing my cool. Then we kiss and remember the love that brought us together in the first place.

I've taken up painting every afternoon as my self-inflicted therapy. I've found this activity centers me the way no other one has. Gardening in the summertime has the same effect. Creating something helps me when times get tough. It's an outlet I need. It could be for you too.

THANKS FOR A QUIET DAY

For the past week we've had temperatures hovering around ninety with humidity in the seventy percent range, and Ken has had a rough patch. Even though our house has central air conditioning, he still experiences weakness from the weather. I express his condition as a bowl full of jelly because he can't control the muscles he needs to sit.

But a change is in the wind — literally. Typically when the weather turns from extreme heat to cooler temperatures, there's always a big storm to follow. Last night produced such a storm. As strange as it seems, we like thunder storms, and we both slept well.

This morning it's gray and still pretty humid, but we're putting our trust in the weatherman who told us the sun is supposed to come out with cooler temperatures. We'll be able to open the windows and go outside on the patio for a hot game of Scrabble.

A good quiet day with a slight breeze is a welcomed relief in many ways.

WHEN DISAPPOINTMENT DARKENS YOUR DOOR

How do you accept disappointments? Do you have a tantrum like a two year old? Do you yell at someone? Or do you swallow the hurt and deal with it another day?

Let's face it. Life usually doesn't fulfill our every expectation. In fact, I have come to the conclusion "life" finds a way to make things harder these days.

Today Ken was supposed to go on an outing, and I had plans to visit a friend I hadn't seen in a couple of weeks. BUT — when I heard Ken hit the bedroom floor, I instantly knew my plans for the day were canceled.

I jumped up to see if he was hurt, and God willing he wasn't. I swear that man has a legion of guardian angels who lay on the floor and break his falls. He rarely hurts himself, and I'm thankful for that, but I also realized we wouldn't be going anywhere today. As soon as I expressed my disappointment like a three-year-old — I hated myself. Here the poor guy is struggling to pull himself up to stand and get into his wheelchair, and I'm cranking about my plans changing. I behaved like a real bitch.

A few days later, I experienced what falling is all about. I leaned over in my office chair to pick a paper from the floor — and WHAM! The chair slid out from underneath me, and I landed on my tail. I struggled to get up, and for at least a week, I felt like a kid who got spanked with the principal's wooden paddle. Every time I sat down, I realized what Ken must experience when he falls. I guess you might say I was enlightened as I got to the bottom of the falling experience. Next time he falls I promise to count to ten before opening my big mouth.

DISCOVERING A NEW CAREER

I graduated college with an English degree with minors in Communication and Women Studies. Because I was an English major, I qualified to teach remedial writing at the local community college. I never wanted to be a teacher, but this opportunity was a new challenge and a tangible check. When one door closes, a window opens.

I taught one class for nine semesters. After three years of this part-time work, I learned I still have no use for students who don't dive into the work and do their best. Another reason for backing away from the front of the room was a hip with degenerative arthritis. I couldn't stand for two or three hours any longer.

After three years of teaching, in my spare time I wrote eight novels. Teaching remedial skills honed my writing and with every successive book my writing improved.

While I was spinning yarns, Ken discovered he has the ability to make "word search" puzzles which we intend to put into a book to raise money for MS.

Spending hours at home day in and day out can be tough; but, with our new activities each day brings us something new. We're creating a new world inside the parameters we've been given. Who knew it would be so fulfilling?

FOREIGN LANDS

I'm exhausted. I've worked all week on financial things I've put on the back burner until they boiled over. I have to be in the right frame of mind to tell creditors why we have fallen behind on our bills. I've also filled out lengthy applications for government programs, including Medicaid, food stamps, and energy assistance.

We've exhausted our retirement money, incurring penalties and taxes because we're too young to take out the money we saved for our "golden" years. Ken's Social Security disability check is spent before it hits our bank account. I don't know what we would do without our friends and family who love us so much. They empathize with our predicament and have come to our rescue with checks and cash when we least expect it.

All I want to know is who would ever dream spiraling into this world of poverty would be so time consuming? I feel like I'm running a small business, completing forms and faxing documents. I truly despise keeping records and filing. It wasn't that long ago

I had a secretary who dealt with this minutia. Like a lot of other chores I've have assumed, this work must be done, and I keep telling myself I'll be a better person for it, and my efforts will help us. I'm just not a believer today.

MAKING CHANGES DOESN'T SOLVE EVERYTHING

After my father died, his estate was settled which gave me a windfall I never anticipated. I've invested my inheritance in remodeling our home to make it safer and more accessible for Ken. The kitchen door was widened by twelve inches. We also planned a built-in table which is high enough so Ken can slide the wheelchair arms under it. I also had the contractors eliminate the half wall and spindles by the front door to make it easier for him to get into the house from outside. We gave the living room a new coat of paint and replaced the carpet with a rug that had a tighter weave and lower pile to stand up under his power wheelchair.

When we finished with the inside renovations, we had enough money to build a new garage, double the size of the patio, and replace the entire driveway. I instructed the contractor to build the garage twice as long as it is wide, so Ken can have a roof over his head whenever he needs to get into the car.

We're enjoying the changes to our home. It's like we've moved, but we didn't have to pack! Now I only wish I could solve Ken's falling problem. I suppose wrapping in bubble wrap is out of the question.

TRAVELING BY PHOTO

My friend Jane sent me photos of her recent trip to Hawaii, and they are so beautiful. The images of lush palm trees and the sparkling sapphire water of the Pacific are a welcomed change to the dreary, gray, wintery weather outside my window.

About twenty years ago, Jane and I saw many beaches in the Caribbean together. It was a fluke we ever met; after all, she lived in Maine, and I lived in Wisconsin. It was lucky our paths crossed through the help of another woman named Robin–who was from the Boston area. We all met on a cruise ship, and we did LOTS of exotic traveling together.

At the time, Jane and Robin were travel agents, and I was just plain lucky. When one of the girls would call and say they were planning to go on a "Fam" trip and asked if I would I like to go along I had nothing holding me back. These excursions came at just the right time—usually before I was ready to pull out my hair because an on-going nasty divorce left me drained.

For the first time in my life, I ignored the practical and responsible side of me. I confessed to being selfish and went on these trips. I learned to snorkel with stingrays, met people from around the country and around the world. Best of all, I could leave my life behind me and laugh with girlfriends for a week. The memories of our adventures will remain in my soul forever. If there should ever be a day when memories fade, I have a volume of great photos to bring them back to life.

As I gaze at Jane's Hawaiian photos, I'm sad Ken and I can't travel anymore. It would be too taxing for him to deal with airports and planes, hotels and unfamiliar beds. When we were first together, we enjoyed many trips. We thought our timeshare property would give us a week of vacation once a year in any place we desired. But even that didn't work out the way we planned.

I've learned to grab opportunities appearing in my path with both hands. I enjoy them and keep the memories close. I've learned waiting for something to happen means it probably won't. There's never a "right" time to make a dream come true.

WHEN RELATIONSHIP
DYNAMICS CHANGE

When a couple faces a progressive disease together, every day brings changes never imagined. The day Ken was diagnosed with MS, I had no idea this disease would change the dynamics of our relationship. As his caretaker, I've become more of a parent than a spouse.

I must make decisions for the two of us because the disease has attacked his frontal lope of the brain. This part of the brain controls judgment and decision making. He also has lesions deep in his brain which controls cognitive skills, emotional expressions, problem solving, and memory. I've witnessed the person I love, morph into a person I barely recognize.

The saddest part of watching my Ken slip away a day at a time is thinking about what it was *supposed* to be. He's ten years younger than I am, so I thought he would be caring for me in my old age. I thought we'd have years of happy retirement, traveling and living out the dreams we set down when we were first married. But a disease we can't control took over and here we are.

Let's face it. I can't sugarcoat this part of what has happened to us. We know we're not alone because many of our friend have slipped into illness at retirement age. Ken and I realize we weren't supposed to live forever, but losing a spouse a day at a time can be harder than a sudden death.

Our choice is to remain positive, enjoying the good days and putting up with the difficult ones. We live every day like it's the last one we'll ever have together. Such phrases have become cliché, but the truth is the truth. And it's a plan which works most of the time.

WHEN WEATHER CALLS
THE SHOTS

It's Saturday–at least that's what television programming tells me. You see, when a person spends most days at home, one day is pretty much like the one before and the one after, so I'm never really sure what day it is.

Today we had planned a road trip to Chicago to celebrate Christmas with Ken's family. But Mother Nature sprinkled snow all night, and we woke to several inches covering the ground. Trying to get to Chicago, which is about a hundred miles away, suddenly got too treacherous to venture outside. Ken's motorized wheelchair doesn't have snow tires or chains, so we will stay at home—again—bummer.

We're both disappointed. Ken's family is so fun, and we hate missing a chance to be with them. There are always lots of laughs, hugs, and positive energy floating around, and we feel good after being with them.

Ordinarily, I just keep the disappointments and heartaches at bay, but today I've grown weary of so many of them. They are definitely something I don't record on my calendar.

A TRIP TO THE GROCERY STORE

I put off going to the grocery store for as long as I could. I'm down to three eggs, a couple cups of milk, and a few canned goods. The freezer is empty. It would be an extreme challenge to try to make a meal out of what I have left. After a week of snow and ice, the weather turned sunny and the temperatures climbed into the mid 30's, so it was a nice day to get the chore done.

Besides the weather challenges, financial challenges have also kept me from going to the grocery store. Ken's Social Security check isn't scheduled to come for another week, so I needed a plan "B". Then an idea popped into my head. I could sell a pair of my gold earrings. At one time, they were my favorites, but as my life stands right now, we need food more than we need gold earrings. The sale gave me the hundred dollars I needed to buy provisions for the week.

The refrigerator filled up quickly with fresh veggies and fruits. The freezer is also stocked with beef, pork, and chicken. I'm so lucky my mother taught me how to cook because I don't have to rely on pricey processed foods. Being able to sauté, braise, stir, and fold allows me to cook from "scratch" which saves a lot of money.

It was a good feeling to see our cupboards and refrigerator full again. I said a silent prayer of thanks because once again, I have what I need. Like the Rolling Stones sang, "You don't always get what you want; you get what you need."

THE CAREGIVING
CHOICE

A SHOCKING PROPOSAL

I believe Ken knew he had MS even before he went through the required battery of diagnostic tests. He had a good idea of the disease progression, but I had to study articles before I really knew what he would face in the coming years.

What surprised me more than anything was the reaction of others when I told them about Ken's diagnosis. More than one person asked me if I was planning to leave him. I was really shocked. I had expected questions, but nothing like that!

As I walked away from such doomsayers, I tried to reason why they would expect me to leave when the going got tough. Did they see a weakness in me? After all, Ken was still mobile at the time. He could get through the day without help. It baffled me why someone would encourage me to walk out on him.

It was the last thing I would do.

Perhaps they had a crystal ball I didn't have. Maybe they knew I would become the bread winner. Maybe they saw all the falls he would take and the disappointments we would share. Maybe they knew poverty would cause us to lose our car and almost our home. But weren't we stronger to face such hardships together?

I think their shocking reaction to my news told me more about them instead of me. Perhaps they had a history of not following through. Perhaps they had experienced something tough they couldn't face. So far—I haven't been given a heavier load than I can carry . . . yet. And that's because so many friends and family have willingly decided to walk this journey with us—with their company, their coins, and their encouragement.

Caregiving is a choice, not a sacrifice.

TRAGEDY BRINGS CHOICES

When I taught English at the community college, I gave my class a writing assignment which required them to discuss how a personal tragedy turned into a strength. Most of them had trouble with the assignment because they couldn't come up with an example. Either they minimized their disappointments or they were too young to have "hit the wall."

If I had to write this assignment, I would tell the story of our marriage. I'd walk my reader through how we've worked together to face several "biggies" with strength and hope.

In 1999, Ken had a seizure in the middle of the night. After several more seizures and a battery of tests, he was diagnosed with epilepsy. The specialist told us if a combination of drugs didn't work, it would mean Ken needed brain surgery. Thankfully, he's been seizure-free for over five years now.

In 2000, Ken was diagnosed with testicle cancer. After a month of setbacks of surgical complications, he had four courses of chemotherapy. I thought I would go to pieces if I ever had to face cancer in anyway, but we each approached the disease as a situation which needed to be managed. He faced the pain and suffering, and I stood by as his advocate.

Our friends stood by both of us with their support. One woman in our church group arranged a committee to transport Ken to his chemo treatments, so I could go to work knowing caring people were with him. His infusions went on for five days, lasting about four hours every day. This course of treatment was done every third week for four months.

After his diagnosis of Multiple Sclerosis in 2006, a neuropsychologist said Ken's memory loss was worse than many Alzheimer's patients she had tested. For the first time in our life together, I cried. Somehow I got through epilepsy and cancer without tears, but this load proved to be too heavy. Once again my dear husband had to face a tough battle, and I wanted to scream and stomp my foot like a two-year-old and yell, "This is not fair!"

When Ken couldn't drive any more, he decided to handle the household chores, so we could have fun weekends. I worried about him being home alone all day, so we bought a lovable Pug and named him Ernie. The arrangement was good for both of them; pugs hate being home alone too.

In 2009 things got really tough. I lost my job, and little did I know this was the beginning of my "retirement." I was too young in years to really retire with parties and fond farewells. Instead, I faded into oblivion. The economy was in the tank, and nobody wanted or needed a person at my middle age. Perhaps the layoff was a blessing in disguise because Ken had progressed to a point where he needed me home all of the time.

Was I ready for my new career as a caregiver? Not really, but then nobody is. Caregiving is something one learns on-the-job.

FRIENDSHIP TILL THE END

The weather this spring has been horrendous. Ken has been cooped up in the house all week, and I don't know how he stays sane. I was lucky enough to escape for a couple of hours to meet girlfriends for lunch while he patiently sits at home, keeping his mind busy with his computer.

Yesterday, though, I got a call from a good friend who needed a ride home from the hospital. Patrick is like a brother to me. For years we've helped each other because we both know we can count on each other. Patrick suffers from Type One Diabetes, and he had to have a toe amputated. He also had angiograms on both legs. So, for three days, he had to stay still for many hours. For him, I think that's worse than being housebound.

I was happy to help Patrick, but Ken wanted to ride along. At first I thought I would have to get Patrick released on my own, but I called his wife, and she went with us. Thank God! I really didn't want the responsibility of taking care of Patrick as well as Ken by myself.

As Linda went into the hospital, Ken and I waited in the car. We both were happy to help Patrick get back home. After Ken couldn't drive any longer, Patrick picked him up every day to have coffee at one of the many coffee shops in our city. Ken joked they solved world problems over a cup of java on a daily basis. Sadly, now both of them are too sick to keep up the tradition.

As we waited, Ken and I talked about how the hospital has grown since he had to be treated there for testicle cancer in 2000. The hospital even provides Valet Parking now. That's BIG TIME! We talked about what we were going to have for supper. Our conversation amounted to nothing, really. But we were out of our four walls sitting in the sun.

Unlike Patrick, Ken doesn't suffer pain with his MS. His day-to-day challenges of fatigue and falling make us lose sight of how much worse his situation could be.

When Linda and Patrick emerged from the hospital and we got everyone situated in the car, the jokes about being in the hospital started to fly. It felt like old times when the four of us met for breakfast every Saturday morning, and we laughed for a couple of hours. Circumstances have changed, but our friendship remains strong. That's all that matters.

Blessings come in small doses, and we're thankful.

WHEN DARKNESS FALLS, LET THE LIGHT IN

As a caretaker, sometimes I find it hard to live in Ken's shadow. It's hard to admit I have challenges, especially when his needs are more immediate and greater than mine.

It's hard to admit I have depression because most people don't understand it. Most people think depression is sadness, but it's so much more than that. It's darkness and sometimes my little flashlight of medication doesn't shine through it. My depression manifests itself in withdrawing. I sit like a lump in my chair and play computer games. I don't even want to write or paint when this happens. Part of the problem is the chemicals in my brain, but the bigger part of it is feeling like such a failure.

I tell myself my life is what I've made it. I do want to stay home and be there for Ken. He struggles so much every day; he also fights depression with medication, but Ken sees the world differently. He never complains because he says doing so would only make me feel bad. He never puts anyone down because he allows people to be who they are. Somehow he keeps himself in a world filled with light.

Yesterday some light came into my darkness. My friend Joyce invited us to have lunch. We first had coffee at her beautiful little home, and then I drove us all to a neighborhood family restaurant for a sandwich. When Ken went to the bathroom, she opened her purse, pulled out a wad of bills and said, "How much do you need?" I knew she was going to help us, but her generosity overwhelmed me. It proved to be one of those rare times I cried. She handed me one hundred dollars. "If you need more, just tell me." Then she hugged me.

Again, God has provided. He does his special work through others, and Ken and I are testimony to His good works. We've benefited in so many ways. The list is long. There is the ramp his aunts and uncles gave us. Then Scott put more work into building it than he originally planned. Jackie and Kay gave me money, so I could buy my books for a book signing. Steve and Tara helped us with the overwhelming drug expense. Ken's Dad paid off the bank, so we could retrieve our car from the impound lot. And now Joyce gave me money to get through another week.

I feel so humbled when all I can do for them is say, "Thank You" with a genuine smile of gratitude. There should be stronger words for such support.

WHEN A WOMAN HAS TO FACE "MEN'S WORK"

Our laundry tubs are clogged. Yuck. I've done what I know what to do and that is get out the Liquid Plumber, pour, and wait—*that's the extent of my plumbing expertise.* I'm sad to say, the chemicals didn't do the trick to clear the clog. After one treatment, the water in the tub drained, but when more water filled the tub it just sat there.

I hate it when household annoyances like this come into my world. Like a lot of women my age, I never learned how to take care of such things—after all, I was raised as a GIRL. Now, I'm just a dumb white collar WOMAN with no household skills other than being able to pound a nail into the wall to hang a picture, or to use a screwdriver to tighten a loose a screw. Oh, and I know how to paint and wallpaper a room.

Now, before you say, "But Barb, you can learn how to do simple household chores." I will tell you that I DON'T WANT TO LEARN. As far as I'm concerned, plumbing expertise is not in my DNA.

I grew up in world where there was a clear line of demarcation between *"men's work"* and *"women's work."* I figure there are just some things I should be left off the hook to fix. I don't do car repairs, and I don't do plumbing and electrical work. Before the last few years, Ken always unclogged pipes and fixed electrical challenges. Now he doesn't have the strength or the cognition to do these things. So, it's up to me to figure out how to get this problem solved.

That's not to say I don't work around the house. You've read about the demarcation of our household chores. So you know I cook, vacuum, load and unload the dishwasher, mop the floors and clean the toilet. I think this is enough.

Getting back to the problem at hand . . . My first instinct was to call a plumber and be done with it. But plumbers make more than CEOs at large corporations, so I needed to come up with another answer. So, I used one of my life lines and phoned a friend. Through the goodness of his heart, Ray stopped over after work to take a look at the problem.

In about an hour, he cleared the clog. Once again a friend rescued us. Thank you, Ray.

EVERY DAY, BE THANKFUL

B eing thankful in tough times is hard. Cold, dark days always puts me in a "down" mood. I'm worn out. I feel trapped and forgotten, and I've given myself a private "pity party" for the past couple of days—even though I know deep in my heart I've chosen to be in this caregiver role.

I'm ashamed to admit this week I've been a bitch. I've been cranky and impatient, and unfortunately Ken is the only person here, so he's on the receiving end of my bad humor. I get tired of waiting as he moves at a snail's pace. I know it's not his fault he moves so slowly, but why do I always have to wait? I want to run away, go on vacation, and forget about my real life.

Thankfully, such episodes don't happen often. And this time, a much needed article about living a thankful life crossed my path and helped me step out of my bad mood.

Let's face it. Moving your mind to a state of being thankful isn't that difficult. I start with the simple things—like being well, like having a warm place to live, like having food on the table, or a buck in my pocket. Even having a reliable old car in the garage which can take me to another place for an hour is a blessing.

My list goes on. Like having a little dog that would rather sit beside me all day than do anything else. Like having a chance to devote my time to writing and painting. Like having a computer to capture my words. Like having a chance to inspire others as a teacher. Like having a host of great friends who love and care about us and are present whenever we need them. If I would continue with this list it would go on for several more pages.

Writing down all of these blessings helps me ditch the "woe is me" feeling. I realize when I'm thankful for what I have, I will never lack anything.

Do I wish things were different? Of course, you see it in most pages of this book, but life brings challenges for everyone. I had dreamed about retiring where the weather is warm in winter and cool in summer. But I chose this life. Opportunities will come and go. Challenges will appear and disappear. I will be happy if I only remember to be thankful. I need to remember that every day.

After all, living thankfully is MAGIC—only it's real!

THE CHALLENGE OF BALANCE

B alance. An important concept in all things from nature to personal health. Throw off the balance, and there will be conflict and trouble.

Trying to achieve and maintain personal balance is as difficult for me as it is for an Olympic gymnast to stay on the balance beam. One slip or bobble to one side or the other can spell disaster.

Trying to keep work, play, and meditation balanced is a constant challenge. If one aspect gets too strong, it pulls on the others. And ta-da! You're in conflict. It makes for a good story, but in real life, being out of balance sucks.

Keeping balance is especially hard when it seems all of the attention in a relationship goes one way. If you're a caregiver, the spotlight rarely shines on you. It focuses on the person in the rela-tionship who needs so much help. Does it mean your needs should be neglected?

If I'm feeling neglected and resentful, it's my fault because I allowed things to get out of whack. I pushed my wishes and needs into the background in the name of being unselfish. Am I really unselfish or am I falling into the martyr trap? The problem lies with me.

It took me several years to realize if I didn't take care of me, I was no good to anyone else. Now I recognize when I need a break. Maybe it's an hour away to spend with a girlfriend. Maybe it's time alone to pamper myself with a soak in the bathtub, or a pedicure at a salon, or even time to get dressed, brush my teeth and comb my hair without an interruption.

I've come to the conclusion in order to achieve success, I have to **work** at something I enjoy (my writing and painting); I have to **play** enough with girlfriends, and I also have to have enough **time alone** to maintain a healthy spiritual life. If I can keep these three important things in balance, happiness and contentment follows.

TRUE LOVE BRINGS THE MOST
AMAZING EXPERIENCES

I f you're still reading, you've realized Ken is an exceptional person. He's kind, gentle, and non-judgmental. He's taught me how to be the same—most of the time. I'm still "in training."

Now that he's finding himself weaker and unable to walk on most days, we're both missing things we used to do together. Not big things. Everyday things. Like shopping and snooping in the antique shops. Like Saturday chores. It always surprises me when I feel a sense of loss when such things don't happen any longer.

I believe we've stayed in step with the deterioration of Multiple Sclerosis which has foisted on us as well as any couple can. He keeps fighting, and I keep supporting. I've learned to be more patient than I ever thought possible. He's learned to be more courageous than he thought possible. Together we face the challenges of the disease never knowing what will be taken away next.

If you have someone in your life who suffers from MS, or Parkinson's or Alzheimer's then you know what I'm talking about.

The first tendency with such a diagnosis is for the healthy partner to run away. I admit I thought about bailing, but then I looked into the eyes of the man I love and knew I could never abandon him.

If you're on the outside looking in, you probably think, "You're married. You have to stay. Remember for better or for worse in the marriage vows?" Let me assure you, it's not an easy decision to make. You know what you should do, but you also wonder if you have the stuff to take on such a heavy load.

Because I decided to stay with Ken for the duration doesn't give me sainthood, but I can attest true love has a powerful effect. Also, making such a decision to become a caretaker doesn't diminish personal needs. Ken understands I need to go off for a couple hours with friends. He always says, "Have a good time, and I'll see you when you get back." He recognizes his illness prohibits me from doing a lot of other things I would like to do. The pendulum swings both ways. It should in a good relationship.

I have no "moral" to this never-ending story, but I would like to tell you if you must face a dire diagnosis, stay the course. There are people who are willing to help, and you will discover things about yourself and your afflicted partner or friend which will amaze you—I can guarantee the experience will bring special moments in your life—just like it has in mine.

KNOCK, KNOCK, KNOCK

Many nights I sleep on the sofa. This is becoming more of a normal occurrence because many nights my arthritic hip seems to need a softer surface than our bed provides. I really don't mind resting on the sofa because I watch television to fall asleep to the "white noise" of a monotone narrator. I actually choose what I watch with that criteria in mind. Ken finds the television keeps him awake, so this is the compromise I made on those sleepless nights which come often.

At 1 a.m. – just a short time after I fell asleep—someone pounded on the door. I sat up and shook the cobwebs from my sleepy head. Flashing red and white lights slipped through the vertical blind, and I quickly realized Ken must have fallen and pressed his life alert button to get some help. Yes, the fire department was once again on our doorstep. I opened the door dressed in my pajamas to four burly men. The good news is they had Ken back into his wheelchair in a couple of minutes and saved the day once again.

I was so shaken by the situation I'm afraid I was not kind. I think my crabbiness with Ken was due to the fact I had just fallen asleep and now I had to clean him up from a failed trip to the bathroom. I hated myself for being cross with him. It wasn't fair to him, but it wasn't fair to me either. He didn't want to get MS, but then again, neither did I.

In thirty minutes, Ken was clean and safely tucked into the bed, and I was alert and wide awake. I had to restart the whole process of getting back to sleep on the sofa. Ernie jumped up into one of the recliners and the house quieted down. After six or so sound hours of slumber, I woke to another thud. I dragged myself up and trudged down to the bathroom to find Ken laying on the floor. Only this time, I was calm and patient.

I'm telling you this as a kind of confession for my bad behavior. I'm also sharing with those of you who might beat yourself up for being cranky with the person you care for. We all have our limits and last night was just too hard. I'm comforted by the fact Ken doesn't hurt himself when he falls because as he says, he relaxes and tries to ease into the effects of gravity. Little does he understand watching him struggle to command his unruly body to move is torture for me too.

All we can do is roll with the situation and ask for a better day. That usually works.

A RUDE AWAKENING

I would imagine some of you who are reading this book haven't experienced what it's like to live with a disabled person. When I decided to write about the day-to-day struggles of a caregiving, I never anticipated it would be this difficult. The last thing I want to do is to make you all feel sorry for me. That is not my intention. I just want to provide a relief value for all the other men and women who are in a similar boat. I want them to know they are not alone. Some people find help in support groups, but I don't. I'm not comfortable talking about private issues with strangers.

If you are one of the lucky ones who has never had to take care of a failing person in your life, perhaps you will understand the challenges other people face and have a bit more empathy for them.

I think of all the thousands of soldiers returning home from the Middle Eastern war with missing legs and arms and traumatic brain injuries. All of them will need help from their wives or parents who overnight get thrown into the role of caregiver. When you love someone more than yourself, caregiving isn't a duty, it's a choice.

I find myself walking a fine line. Sometimes I do too much. Sometimes I feel I don't do enough. The last thing I want to do is take away Ken's personal power. We have discussed this balancing act, and Ken has asked me to stand back and allow him to try to take care of himself. This is tough because I'm a fixer. I'm also impatient. What takes him an hour I can do in a few minutes, but he deserves a chance to try. This has been a difficult lesson to learn.

This morning Ken struggled to get out of bed and crashed on the hardwood floor. Again I was jolted from a sound asleep. I asked if he was hurt; he replied No," but he wanted to rest on the floor before trying to get up. Watching him lie there was hell.

I let the dog out, made coffee, and fed the cat his morning treat of wet food. Then I went back into the bedroom to aid Ken. I witnessed him trying to get back on his feet. He turned and twisted without much progress. I asked him if I should call for help, and he said no; he wanted to keep trying.

During the next ten minutes I watched his determination propel himself into his wheelchair. Now all we had to do was change his disposable underwear. Yeah. That's part of his care too — to change him when he has accidents. Most people cringe when I talk about such things, but cleaning up messes of all kinds fall into an unwritten job description.

The good news is Ken didn't hurt himself. He may have a bruised butt, but his determination to keep trying is heroism in my book.

AN "EASEL" ESCAPE

The weather hasn't gotten any warmer, so it's another day inside. After taking care of Ken's breakfast needs, writing a piece for my blog, watching a favorite television show, I found myself in front of my easel once again.

I've never taken a drawing or painting class, but my artist friend Marie has taken me under her wing and agreed to teach me. I try to absorb all her tutorage, and over the past couple of years I have improved.

My painting didn't turn out very well today, but that's okay. Having a creative outlet to let my mind wander is almost as good as a vacation. For an hour or two, I can leave my life and escape to a world that is different every day. I let my imagination fly and sometimes I produce a good painting, more often I don't. But it doesn't matter.

Caretakers need outlets to ward off the overwhelming responsibility they must undertake. Thinking for someone beside yourself is tough work, and I've found these little daily escapes with a paintbrush in my hand feeds my soul. It helps me greet a bad day with the love and attention Ken deserves.

AM I WAITING FOR GODOT?

I feel a little like a character in the famous play, *"Waiting for Godot,"* by Samuel Becket. Lately, like Estragon or Vladimir, I feel I'm basically living the same day over and over again. My past life of travel and new explorations are over, and here I am waiting all of the time.

My usual rosy disposition has taken a downturn today because Ken is moving more slowly than usual. I need to wait for him no matter what we have to do. His walking is tenuous, and I hold my breath he doesn't fall. When our friend Patrick joins us, I have to wait for the two of them, running ahead to open doors.

Now I have to add my elderly father to the mix. My sister has done the heavy lifting as his health fails at age 89. I have been waiting for the "next shoe to fall" as he lays in the hospital. And the waiting goes on and on.

I wait for the UPS guy to deliver my latest novel. I wait for inspiration to come for a new post daily for my blog. I'm also waiting for my editor to get back to me about my novel in progress. And so it goes.

Am I really living a life like in the play where nothing really happens, but yet audiences stay glued to their seats?

The characters Estragon or Vladimir drag themselves through nothingness, keeping the audience guessing about the point of the play. Does life have no meaning? But time changes each character, and what are these two men really waiting for?

Perhaps the point is the true joy in life is in the waiting to see what each day brings. If a person simply walks through life without a purpose, he will be waiting a long time. The present is all any of us have. We can either rejoice in having another day, or let the day slip by waiting for something better. You have to choose.

Living in the past is fruitless; living in the future is tenuous, but living in the here and now is after all, a "present."

WHAT DAY IS IT, ANYHOW?

"I wouldn't know what day it is, if I didn't take pills."
Yup, that was the first thing Ken said this morning. It was one of those small things which puts the larger picture in focus. Being home has suspended the outside world in certain ways. Knowing what day it is has become more important to him. Interesting isn't it?

I've talked about time before, but to me time is such an interesting concept. It changes with age and circumstance. When you're young and have the world by the tail, time seems infinite. An alarm clock wakes you to get ready for work. You go through a morning routine and drive to your destination. If you have a desk, there's a calendar sitting there, showing you what day it is. If you don't have a desk, there are certain activities you must do in a given day. Time is measured very differently when you stay home every day.

When we all lived on farms, knowing what day it was wasn't important. People worked from sun-up to sun-down. Arriving a few minutes late didn't mean we'd be "written-up" by a supervisor.

Measuring time came during the industrial revolution. Factories and offices had to run on schedule to fulfill orders and get goods to market on time. Days of the week, hours, and minutes became more important to keep things moving in an orderly fashion.

Believe me, I don't miss being jarred from sleep by some digital nuisance. I don't miss fighting traffic and construction work on the highways. But being home with Ken has forced us to consult an outside source to just know what day it is or we can simply take our pills which are waiting for us in a weekly pill sorter.

THE RECEIVING END OF
CARE GIVING

B efore lunch today, a nasty virus hit me. Somewhere between the pharmacy and the grocery store the nasty beast invaded my body. I retreated to the living room sofa interrupted by the need to make frequent trips down the hall to the bathroom. Headache, body aches, fever, and digestive problems flattened me for a day. I can attest I haven't been this sick since I had a ruptured appendix. The hardest thing for me to do is to stay still and let the virus run its nasty course.

My spirit still wanted to prepare dinner, but my weak body held me back. I couldn't help Ken the way I'm so used to preparing meals, which now means cutting everything into bite size pieces because the tremors in his arms make the cutting motion difficult. When I can't take care of him like I normally do, I feel a sense of failure – even though logically I know I'm temporarily out of commission.

He's a trooper, though. It's one of the reasons I love him so much. He stayed by my side quietly working on his computer asking me periodically if there is something he could get for me.

My short escapade into the world of the sick made me realize receiving caregiving is just as hard as giving it.

⊫+⊨

The nasty virus which attacked me on Friday has taken a step back. Thank goodness! I'm not up to full power, but 85% is pretty good. We finally got a break in the hot weather, but the cool temps came with rain and dreary, gray skies.

Ken did his best to take care of me by fetching water and pills. He scrounged his meals from leftovers he could microwave. It was strange to have our roles reversed. But that's Ken. He's always put me first in our relationship, and I do believe that's very special.

Unfortunately, after I was well enough to vacate the sofa for good, I found piles of messes. Ken can't help it for two reasons — one he's not able to keep things neat because his disability doesn't allow too much leeway and two, he's a man who doesn't think of such things.

So today, I'll tackle the dishes in the sink, and I'll put away open cans and boxes of stuff he used to keep going when I was sick. What I want to know is: *Where's that fairy godmother when I need one?*

FRIENDS AND FAMILY TO THE RESCUE

WOMEN AND FRIENDSHIPS

I never knew how to be a friend when I was a child. I lived on a block over populated with boys, so I learned how to ice skate, throw and catch a baseball, climb trees and other activities boys do. I was fourteen when I learned what it took to be a good girlfriend when Debbie came into my life. We got closer than sisters through our teenage years and into adulthood sharing disappointments and happiness.

Through the years our friendship faded with husbands, children, and jobs. It wasn't until just recently we connected. We didn't really have to "catch up" to have a good conversation, but we did talk about what our kids were doing, where they lived, and other day-to-day happenings.

Debbie gave me a rare gift so many years ago. She showed me what it took to be a good friend, and since then I have put her teachings to good use and made other wonderful friends along the way. I'm happy to say my best friend is Ken, but I also have filled my life with girlfriends who enrich and fill my life.

My friend Kay moved to Florida about a year ago and now we talk on the phone at least once a week, but it's not the same as being together. In a few days I'm flying down to see her. We didn't plan anything for our time together; in fact I'll be content to sleep late and not be responsible for anything. Our time together will amount to a number of hours, but when it's time to say goodbye with a hug, we'll feel lighter, happier and thankful we had a good visit. It's like we both need an infusion of each other. It's something our husbands can't provide.

Being with Kay reinforces something I've always felt–there's nothing as important to a woman as her friendships. Women NEED girlfriends. And if I'm lucky, I'll maintain a whole stable of relationships with other women who will carry me through from girlhood to the grave. "Girl's Days" of shopping, conversations over a cup of coffee, even a short talk over the backyard fence are all important events to most women. We seem to need this connection with one another.

I guess it figures these relationships are at the heart of my stories and novels. When men are gone and children leave, girlfriends stay. Friendships are essential to my life. I always am grateful for the women who have come into my life and who have chosen to stay. They are like gifts I never expected to receive.

RECONNECTING WITH A COLLEAGUE

Ken's well enough to leave him for an hour or two on the good days, so today I met a friend for a cup of coffee. Boyd and I were associates at Met Life about five years ago; in fact, I helped train him. We met in college almost twenty years before that when we were both involved in the student government. After graduation, he became a political organizer, and I went into marketing communications where I spent twenty years in project management.

We both found ourselves in the insurance industry after leaving the careers we loved but couldn't find work. Now both of us are caretakers. A terrible fall left his wife with profound disabilities, and now he assumes most of the domestic responsibilities like me.

Boyd and I enjoyed our little respite from our "real" lives. Our short visit gave us both a chance to laugh and catch up. I think we both left a little lighter than when we first sat down. Our visit was good for both of us.

Short, impromptu outings give me just enough of a break to face the rest of the day in good spirits. I value these times like gold.

WHEN FRIENDS RESURRECT

When you find you're the person who must take care of another, sometimes you get stuck—at least I do. I feel paralyzed when I need to make decisions for another adult. Thinking for two is hard work but it is necessary. I realized I had to accompany Ken on all of his doctor visits because he has a tendency to make up stories when he can't remember how things have transpired.

Just when I thought I might go crazy, a long lost friend entered my life again. She had been her mother's caretaker for over five years. Her mother suffers from Alzheimer's, and Pam has been down this caregiving road before me. She knows all the pot holes. She commiserated with me, listened to my challenges and pointed me in the right direction to get help.

She told me about an organization called the Aging and Disability Resource Center. She said there were many professionals there who could make my life easier and I should give them a call.

The hardest thing for me was to pick up the phone. I was put in touch with the Caregiver Support Manager, and she put me in touch with other people in the organization who could give us help. Sharing my story with a friend made all the difference. I never realized the ADRC could help solve my problems.

TRUE LOVE SHOWS UP
ON VALENTINE'S

I've come from the depths of despair to be revived by my dear friends and my beautiful in-laws who have once again surrounded us with their love. It's painful to publicly discuss this catastrophe, but the outcome was beautiful.

I just want you to understand, Ken and I always paid our bills on time and maintained an excellent credit rating, that is, until this year when we only had his Social Security check to live on, and I can't seem to buy a job. We hit rock bottom when we found the repo man in our driveway. Our car was repossessed.

After Ken and I got our belongings out of the car, I handed the tow truck driver my keys. I didn't cry. Instead, I went into the house and sat on a kitchen chair feeling numb. It was almost as if this horrible, humiliating thing had just happened to someone else. That evening, Ken sat beside me, and put his arm around me. We didn't say a word but we each were wondering how our lives had gone so wrong.

After a couple of hours of accepting what had happened, I found enough strength to call friends. Ken called his parents. Before we knew it, we were surrounded in love.

"It'll be all right, Barb." They all said. Then they took action.

By the next day, Ken's father went to the bank and paid off the balance of our loan. My other friend, Jackie gave me money to get the car off the impound lot. Terry brought me the reflux medicine I needed and took with me to the impound lot where our car was being held hostage. When I returned home, Kay told she's going to spearhead some kind of fund raiser to help us.

The moral to this very personal story is this: *Friends and loving parents are the greatest gifts the Universe gives us.* This Valentine's Day love was expressed in its truest form. Not with roses. Not with candy. Just with unconditional love from our friends and family.

THE EVIDENCE OF ANGELS
IN ACTION

Today I'm listening to the buzz of a saw, the popping of a nail gun, and the rattle of a steel tape measure. Yes, we have some construction going on at our house. Scott our contractor and his associate are building a wheelchair ramp for Ken. Our project developed by the grace of Ken's extended family.

The project started a couple of months ago, when we were touched by an angel. Aunt Lil took it upon herself to organize an effort to help her nephew, "Kenny." Through her research and fund raising, my husband Ken is getting what he needs to be able to easily get out of the house in his power chair.

Aunt Lil and her brother, Uncle Donnie, another member in Mom McCloskey's family of thirteen, took action on this project. Most of the brothers and sisters live in a small Illinois town where they grew up, and everyone I have met has been warm and genuine. The monetary help they have given us can only be repaid with gratitude and thanks, and now we have a monument going up which is tangible proof of their generosity.

I'm not a religious person, but I am spiritual, and I recognize when God has touched other souls to come to the aid of one in need. That's what is really happening here. I am in awe of what the power of love can accomplish.

ANGELS IN THE FLESH

Going through an experience like MS is a journey which can be perilous. Somedays the road is clear of traffic and some days you find yourself in a log jam. Financially, MS will put you in a pit. It's one of my biggest frustrations – not having enough money to do the "normal" things.

But every once in a while, I see light at the end of the never-ending tunnel. This week was like that. God sent me a flock of angels.

Last week, I came up short to buy my medication. Two days later at the grocery store, I also came up short at the cash register. Part of me wanted to cry right there in front of the line of people who had queued up behind me. I truly thought I had enough money left on my food stamp card to cover most of my purchases and the few pennies I had in my bank account two days ago should have covered the rest.

But alas, I was wrong. I began eliminating items from my cart to get down to the bare essentials, only to find I was still ten dollars short. Behind me I could feel the other customers growing impatient because I was holding up the line. Needless to say, I was ashamed and embarrassed.

The lady behind me pulled out a ten dollar bill and handed it to the clerk. Then she turned to me and said, "Please let me help you. It is my pleasure. I believe in paying it forward." Now I really wanted to cry, but not from embarrassment, but from gratefulness. This stranger reached out to me and offered a generous gift. Who was I not to accept it?

And the kindness didn't stop there. In the afternoon, the lady from the IRIS Medicaid program came by for a meeting with good news. Ken received an enrollment date of June 2nd to enter the program. I also had been approved as his caretaker. What this means is the State of Wisconsin will pay me to take care of him—something I've been doing for over three years for free because I deeply love my husband. The extra money will help us stay in our house, and his state insurance will cover his medical expenses. Talk about manna falling from heaven!

But wait! I'm not through yet. Yesterday, another angel crossed my path with a gift. One of my dearest friends read the account about my inability to buy my medication, and she handed me money to cover the cost. This time, I did burst into tears.

The morale of the story is God does hear your prayers. According to the Christian Bible, Jesus told us, "Ask and you shall receive." He wasn't lying. What most people do not realize is God (or the Universe or a Higher Power) works through people. When you get an offer of help from a friend, a family member or even a stranger, accept it and realize your prayers are answered. If you don't believe in God, then know if you think about something hard enough, you will manifest it into your life. It's the law of attraction—it's as real as gravity.

THERE ARE
GOOD TIMES

SAVORING A MOMENT

During the last few years, I've discovered when life boils down from the excitement of youth, it's the simmering of adulthood which makes things tender and produces the best flavor.

The planets must have aligned because the day proved to be perfect. Bright sunshine replaced the winter's usual gray. The remaining snow melted, and the pavement dried. The usual January frigid temperatures warmed into the 40s. Hemmingway always said not to ignore the weather in your story—really, he did say that.

Best of all, Ken felt energetic and well enough to venture out. It was a day for celebration! We jumped in the car, got much needed haircuts, and treated ourselves to lunch at a nice restaurant with one of our Christmas gift certificates.

It had been a couple of months since we were able to sit in a restaurant and smile across the table at each other. I know he was thinking such an occurrence used to be "normal." Even ordinary. But now sitting in a restaurant is special because it's so rare.

Ken joked with the waitress, while she served us. We stuffed ourselves on mussels, salad, and bread sticks as we saw each other from a different perspective. We were on a "date." It even felt romantic. (I'm sure this seems rather curious for two middle-aged people who are together 24/7, doesn't it?)

Ken's Multiple Sclerosis and all its nasty traits took a vacation today, so we enjoyed a break in our daily monotony. We enjoyed the waitress catering to us as Italian music wafted in the background. We listened to the buzz of the other patrons as we laughed together. We even held hands across the table.

All too soon it was time to leave. Our adventure lasted ninety minutes, but those ninety minutes will sustain us for many days. What a wonderful day!

SPENDING A PERFECT DAY

I love sunshine, blue skies, and warm temperatures, but during a Wisconsin winter such a day is a rarity. The weatherman is predicting rain and snow for tomorrow, so yeah, winter isn't done with us yet.

Like most mornings, Ken is weak on his feet, but he was able to pour himself a bowl of cereal, a cup of juice and coffee, peel an orange—all without waking me.

In the afternoon, we went to the gas station, so I could learn how to air up my front left tire, which looks a bit too flat. I know it sounds ridiculous but doing car stuff intimidates me as much as cutting grass and other "man" chores. I still haven't grown accustomed to my changing role.

Because we had no real plans to do anything but air up the tire, we told Ernie he could ride along. Of course, like most dogs, he is always thrilled to "go for a ride." He sits on a pillow perched on Ken's lap with his ears back, and like the Red Barron, he's ready for anything.

After going to a couple of gas stations, we finally found a working air machine. I plunked in two quarters and voila! We had air.

Ken supervised from the front seat, while I removed the cap on the tire valve and placed the air hose in position to put a few pounds into the squishy tire. As I went through the motions of filling the tire, I felt so foolish to have been afraid of something so simple. In two minutes, we were on our way again with Ken praising me for doing such a good job.

To celebrate my great victory, we stopped in to see friends who welcomed us to come in for a visit. Heidi made lattes, and we sat and laughed for a couple hours about my escapade with the tire (and lots of other topics). We left around six o'clock to go home for dinner.

Ken was able to walk sure-footed into the house with his walker; Ernie had behaved himself like the "perfect" dog the entire time, and I was happy knowing we can just pop in on good friends unannounced and be so beautifully welcomed.

THE POWER OF AN ICE
CREAM CONE

It's eighty degrees early in May. The sky is blue. The birds are singing. (Cue the harps.) Seriously, it is a gorgeous day. It was a perfect day to drive our friends Dave and Terry to the airport with the car windows open.

Ken didn't want to ride along because he said he was feeling "under the weather." I insisted he come because he'd been in the house all week, and I thought a change of scenery might cheer him up. He finally gave in and pouted in the passenger's seat. He changed his frown to a smile when Dave and Terry got in the back seat. It appeared my logic worked.

Because extreme weather fluctuations are normal in Wisconsin, I knew I had to seize this day to have some fun. I wanted Ken to enjoy the day with me. I'll admit it. My motives were selfish. I wanted some time with him away from our four walls. I know he felt crappy because he's always up for an outing, but I also know the power of seeing friends energizes him. Besides, I had a surprise in mind for him.

After we wished our friends a good journey, I rolled the windows down, turned up the radio and blasted out of the airport. I headed north–the opposite direction from going home. I had a plan I hoped would perk up my sweet husband, so I headed for "Leon's" – his favorite frozen custard place in Milwaukee.

As we drove along, Ken didn't say anything. Now, I was really worried about him because he always comments when I take a different route–especially one in the opposite direction of where we should be going. It wasn't until he saw St. Luke's hospital in the distance, he realized where he was.

He grinned like a little boy. "We're going to that ice cream place, aren't we?"

I smiled." It's about time you figured out where we are. Yes. I thought you'd like a treat."

I pulled into the nostalgic ice cream shop dating back to the 1940s, parked the car, and walked up to the window to place our order for two double-dip cones.

With a big broad smile, I handed him his favorite butter pecan treat, and we sat in the parking lot, enjoying every lick. As we quietly pretended it was summer, we chatted about how good the ice cream was. We talked about dinner options. We both hoped Dave and Terry would have a good time on their vacation. For about ten minutes, we were our old selves. For those few minutes MS vanished. All because of a simple treat.

After the last lick, I started the car and blended into the heavy 27th Street traffic. As I drove along, I turned up the oldies on the radio and sang along. I felt like a teenager. Ken smiled as I belted out, "Born to Be Wild." Our little excursion turned out to be magical. Not only did Leon's lifted Ken's spirits, it brought me back to some of the happiest, most carefree times in my life. Singing the tunes I loved as a teenager made me feel young and carefree.

Simple pleasures are there for the taking. Enjoying an ice cream cone in the middle of the week, getting out into the good weather, and belting out the "oldies" produced smiles and laughter. Best of all the happiness lingered for the next few days.

We've learned not to wait for "special" occasions because such times are rare. *Carpe diem–Baby!*

YOU GET WHAT YOU ASK FOR

I t's going to be a good day. The sun is shining, the sky is blue, and temperatures are in the low 70s. But that's not why I know it will be a good day– but it certainly helps.

How do I know that? Because I think it will be a good day. It's as simple as that. **Believing** it will be a good day is a self-fulfilling prophesy.

No matter the circumstance, healthy or ill, rich or poor, young or old–we all create our own world. Isn't that great to know?

I know. You're thinking I'm putting on my Pollyanna cloak, but I'm not. I've learned if I think positively and believe I'm going to have a wonderful day, I will. It doesn't matter if I'm going outside my home or just staying in. I will find happiness because I demand it.

Conversely, if I'm tired and crabby and negative, I may as well go back to bed because I certainly will have a bad day. I confess every once in a very long while, I want to be cranky and have a pity party. I'm human after all. But thank goodness, I never dwell on negative thoughts for too long.

I think we all have a responsibility to live a life that is full of wonderful days. So drink your coffee, go through your morning routine, and then face the world with a smile.

It works. Believe me.

COMPUTER-AIDED GIFT GIVING

My birthday is on Friday. Since Ken lost his driving privileges, he always feels a sense of remorse when he can't go to the store and buy me a "just right" present. I miss his thoughtfulness and uncanny ability to *ALWAYS* buy me a gift I love. We've both accepted the loss of his shopping expertise as just one more challenge in our journey through the world of MS.

Everybody asks me what I'd like for my special day, but I have most everything I need. Don't misunderstand. I love presents and surprises, but I don't like asking for specific gifts. However, my present laptop is over six years old and I've had to duct tape the one side of it, so I asked for a new a new laptop.

Like an answer from the gods, I got an email from Dell. It turns out they are having a sale, so I asked Ken if he'd like to give me a new laptop for my birthday. He smiled. Getting a new laptop was a good solution, seeing he got a new dishwasher for his birthday, so I ordered a new computer.

Not only did I get a wonderful low price on the machine of my choice, they offered a free update to Windows 10, a fifty dollar instant rebate, and free overnight shipping. I think Dell knew it was my birthday, too!

A COMING TOGETHER
OVER WORDS

Ken is feeling well today, so we met over a Scrabble board this afternoon. We have a long history playing this game. In fact our love was sealed when he beat me at my favorite game on our first date. I had to insist on a rematch because *NOBODY* ever beat me at Scrabble! I teased him it was a sneaky way of assuring himself a second date.

That second date turned into a lifetime of great fun. Scrabble has been one of the glues which has held us together. We play this word game so much we invested in a "travel Scrabble" board and tiles.

We always played the game on vacation at our timeshare. In fact, the game has traveled with us through the Caribbean, Mexico, Panama, Aruba, Florida, Arizona, on land and sea. Well, you understand. We both are nerds at heart.

Now we play at restaurants or coffee shops. Somebody usually stops by our table and asks who's winning. To us, who wins really doesn't matter because we are so equally matched. We kept a log of wins and losses for over three years and the tally showed we were tied for number of games won.

Luckily, Scrabble is one passion we still have. Our travel vacations are over, but now we challenge each other at the dining room table or when the weather's nice, you can find us on the patio underneath a colorful umbrella counting up the score.

We find joy in in simple things. Scrabble is just one of them.

MAKING A CHOICE – DRAMA OR THANKFULNESS?

Yesterday was about as perfect as it gets. For some people the simple events of taking a drive, doing a little shopping, having lunch with a good friend, and driving home would be taken for granted as an ordinary day. But when you face the daily rigors of caretaking having a relaxing day with a friend becomes a terrific outing. Remember perspective and living a thankful life?

Lately, there has been so much talk about living a "thankful" life. Some therapists even suggest keeping a thankful diary. Why? It is a way to recognize how wonderful a simple life can be. When you're thankful, you don't worry about what you don't have.

Many people sleepwalk through their lives and slug their way through the day. They go through unnecessary drama and whirl around to get attention. Little do they realize they are only wasting precious energy. I would hate living in such a world, so I work to avoid it.

I've shared some of the bad days Ken has experienced, and I admit his deteriorating condition affects me. The bad days are hard, and that's because I love him. But most of the time we work through the challenges together and go on. Through the twenty years we've been together we've become part of each other. Every day I search for ways to make his life easier and happier. Other people look at us staying at home almost every day and wonder why we aren't nuts. After all, this 24/7 togetherness even for healthy people can be enough to make you go crazy.

We've had to accept our retirement dreams are dashed, but our story is much more prevalent than people realize. Our friends are examples of couples who face similar challenges every day. Cathy nurses Jim who has a rare blood disease. Linda watched Patrick lie in a hospital bed for a few months before he succumbed to the ravages of diabetes. Kay has seen her husband Marc collapse with diabetes and heart disease. We all muddle through the tough days and give thanks for days when our partner feels well. The only other choice is to run away, but that isn't a true option. None of us could live with ourselves if we gave into that impulse.

Being thankful for the good things keeps the awful days in perspective. And believe me, there are many awful days. But discovering the peace that exists inside helps me take the disappointments in stride. When a I found my personal peace, I can dismiss the small stuff. Before you realize it, everything is the small stuff.

A DAY SPENT ALONE

Yesterday I spent the late morning and early afternoon alone. Ken went on an outing. He felt well. Even though everyone in the group is decades older than him, Ken has made friends in this group. He loves visiting with older people.

Usually I spend these four or five free hours with my friends, today I chose to be alone. I hunted new winter tops at the thrift store. At first the store was a necessity, now it a preference. I love a good bargain! Then I went home and ate lunch with Ernie sitting on my lap. He watches every bite go into my mouth, hoping I might share a bite with him. I enjoyed my soap opera without somebody teasing me for watching such drivel, and I didn't talk for four hours! Believe me, that's a record!

When I picked up Ken at 3:30 p.m., we both looked forward to being together again. With stuffed peppers and acorn squash waiting in the oven, we had a pleasant dinner as we talked about the day's events.

After dinner, we cleared the dishes and settled in for a night of television. In the past, days like this would have bored me to death, but as I have said many times we cherish these mundane times. Achieving normalcy in our world is what we strive for because we both realize someday we won't be able to be together. We want to put that day as far into the future as we can.

OTHER
THOUGHTS

GRAY DAYS ARE GOOD FOR SOMETHING

I hate Wisconsin winters. Even though the scene outside the window is pristine with a white blanket of snow covering the ugliness of dead grass, and ice clinging to branches like Waterford crystal, there is danger lurking under the beauty. Mother Nature is a cagey one. She lulls us into a state of wonder . . . and then Wham! Reality strikes. Lift that shovel! Balance on that ice! Worst of all, the beauty doesn't last long. In a few days, a dirty residue will cover everything.

I've come to the conclusion winter is for children. I remember days when I'd play with the neighborhood kids, having snowball fights, building snowmen, and sliding down hills on sleds all day long. And then of course, winter is also for those grown-up children who enjoy scooting from bar to bar on their snowmobiles. There are still others who look forward to taking their lives in their hands as they tear down the slopes on two skinny skis. But for Ken and I, the gray days of the winter months are spent indoors looking at each other.

On top of that, January means it's time to take down the Christmas decorations. I left them up until Ken's parents came up from Chicago, but that was just an excuse. They visited during the day, so the lights weren't turned on.

Today, I'm mourning as I stash away water-proof pine garland, strings of lights and my outdoor five foot lighted angel, all of which will hibernate in the garage until they will shine next year. The process inside the house is the same. I strip the living room of all the colorful lights and bobbles and pack the Christmas tree in its box to store in the basement. As I look at the bare surroundings, I feel like something beautiful died.

A person would think by now this "reverse decorating" process would be normal, but every year is the same for me. The soft twinkle of holiday lights is replaced by darkness and cold temperatures which make me long for a warm summer day.

THE WONDER OF STARS

Ken and I enjoy the Science Channel. I think I'm intrigued because when I was younger I was intimidated by the discipline. How dumb was that? I am so sorry I let my fear of the unknown drive me away from science. As I watch the interesting programs on the Science Channel, I realize what I missed. Too bad. Perhaps my childhood fascination with the planets and stars might have turned me into an astronomer—but then I would have had to get over my math phobia, too.

Last night we learned *EVERYTHING* in the universe is part of the *STARS*, and that includes us! Wow! Think about it! The energy, matter, water, and minerals we are made of came from outer space! *WE* are a product of the amazing universe! ***We Really Are Star People!***

Of course, it took billions of years to make planet Earth. First space dust from an exploding star had to attract by static electricity. Then those dust balls formed asteroids, and as the asteroids clunked into each other, they bound together. When they got big enough, gravity took over and then there was a few more billion years for the comets to come along to crash into earth and provide water—the stuff of life. Then a few more billion years and humans appeared on the scene. But think of it! How great is it to know we are all part of the vast universe in which we live.

I wish everyone on the planet could have seen that program. If we all saw ourselves as part of a great universe, we might even think twice before putting another person down for being different. If we embraced our differences, we might realize we are more alike than different because we come from the same place.

I'm thinking about these things because I watch people relate to Ken differently now that he is in a power wheelchair. People either ignore him or over-compensate speaking in high voices like a person does when talking to a baby. He accepts their behavior. I find it more difficult to overlook their ignorance.

I guess the old adage applies: *Do on to other as you would have them do to you.* Yeah. That works. After all, we are star people who should shine together.

WARNING! — A "HUGGER" IS ON THE LOOSE!

I confess. I'm a "hugger." Yeah, I'm a gregarious person who reaches out and hugs people. Whether I'm saying "hello" or "goodbye," if you're in my world, you'll probably get a hug from me. You see, I believe most of us suffer from "hug deprivation." I've made hugging my personal quest, especially now because Ken is unable to hug me very often.

I attribute my "hugginess" to my Italian heritage. When I was a child, I was expected to greet my aunts and uncles with a kiss and a hug when we entered their homes; we also were expected to repeat the process when we left. As teenagers, we were embarrassed, but a hug didn't kill us, after all hugs were signs of love and respect.

Hugging is a basic human need. Our skin is our antenna which "feels" love through hugging. We feel acceptance. Believe it or not, hugging promotes good chemicals which save us from ill health. Everyone needs hugs, and I'm not just talking through my liberal, touchy-feely self, either. Here's a list I edited from _Kathleen Keating_ "Hug Therapy":

- Hugs feel good.
- Hugs cure loneliness and depression.
- Hugs help overcome fear.
- Hugs open doors to feelings
- Hugs builds self-esteem.
- Hugs slow down aging (huggers stay younger longer)
- Hugs ease tension.
- Hugs affirm a connection with another human being.

That's a pretty long list, wouldn't you say?

I miss Ken's hugs more than I can tell you. His balance issues get in the way of standing and hugging each other like we used to do. Now our infrequent hugs have taken on more significance. These rare times solidify why we are still together for better or for worse.

A TOUCH OF BEAUTY

I t snowed last night. Just an inch or two—enough for the snow
plow guys to show up and charge us fifty bucks. I try not to think
about the cost as the snow falls. In our situation, we need help with
this burdensome winter chore. Instead, I'm looking out my window and enjoying the scenery. I see a confectionery dusting over
sleepy tree limbs and bare bushes. It's truly beautiful. On days like
this, I'm thankful I can stay home, sip my coffee, and watch the
stillness outside the window.

I notice the red, white and blue of an American flag waving in
contrast to the grayness of the cold day. The banner gently floats
from a flagpole in the cemetery across the street.

As I watch the flag, I think some people are like that flag. In
their quiet way, they can't help draw attention to themselves just
because they are so beautiful. Like my husband Ken. In his own
quiet way, he goes on without complaining about his everyday challenges. Like the flag, he bears the injustice of looks and stares
because he stands out without trying.

True beauty goes deep. I'm not talking about physical beauty.
Let's face it; some of the most beautiful faces are true beasts under

the make-up! What I'm talking about is a quiet beauty in caring eyes and gentle voices. A keen sense of humor makes people giggle on really bad days. Somehow their mere presence makes a difference. Such people are everyday heroes going on about their lives, unknowingly touching others in profound ways.

People are drawn to putting such a person in their realm. Once they decide to be your friend, you never let them go. Like that flag, they bring a touch of beauty into an otherwise dreary existence. We are all lucky they walk the earth. I know. I live with a beautiful person who has lavished me with unselfish love and happiness for over twenty years.

PRIME TIME FOR PRIMROSES

When I was in the grocery store yesterday heading down the home stretch to the check-out station, a beautiful little plant called to me. It was a pink and yellow Primrose.

I have always had a soft spot for these dainty little flowers because they are the first signal spring is just around the corner. *Right.* It's January in Wisconsin. Who am I kidding? This far north, winter has been known to stretch well into the month of May!

The plant was marked ninety-nine cents, so I picked it up and brought it home. I planted the perky little plant in a pretty little fluted vase and set it on my kitchen table. For some reason, I smile every time I look at its lush green leaves and sweet little pink flowers. I tell the plant she's beautiful.

I enjoy the sweet little flowers as long as they will last. You see, our house is a plant killing zone. With the houses so close and big pine trees in the yard, I have no good place to give plants what they need—sunlight—direct or otherwise. The best I can do is pray this sweet little beauty will be strong enough to live until I can safely plant her outside.

Ken knows how many times my indoor gardening efforts have failed, and he just smiles at my persistence. I think deep down inside he's praying this little plant will make it until April because it's brought me so much joy on a day when the wind chill temperature is 25 degrees *BELOW* zero.

I think having flowering spring plants in the house during the dead of winter is a kind of therapy. The perky blooms blossom in the face of the cold offer a quick cure for the cabin fever. So when you see primroses or daffodils smiling at you in the grocery store, rescue them with your love. You both will be better for it.

A FAST WEEK

This week has sped by faster than most. I find this curious because Ken and my daily schedule runs on a pretty regimented track. But I've always found "time" to be an interesting concept. Neanderthals or the early Homo sapiens probably never had time affect them the same way it does us. Instead of chasing deadlines, they were consciously trying to stay alive and not be eaten by a saber-tooth tiger or some other beast.

I understand there are scientific reasons why time behaves the way it does, and it's an interesting topic for novels–specially science fiction stuff, but I see time as a *finite* quality to be used wisely.

Maybe time went fast this week because I found the energy to do things I've been putting off for quite awhile. I can't tell you what precipitated the change from a slothful lump to a ball of fire, but I did things like get the tax papers together, call numerous agencies for one reason or another, make appointments with doctors and arrange payments with creditors. Balancing these taxing realities, required I take time to create a painting, add a few chapters for the next novel, and meet a caregiving counselor at the Aging and Disability Resource Center (ADRC).

The latter was the hardest of all because I finally accepted the fact I wanted help. Admitting I needed help was hardest of all because it meant defeat. I felt weak and pathetic as I waited for my appointment to begin. All of my life I have put on a façade of strength and confidence, so showing human weakness is humiliating for me.

Ken struggled terribly for the last two weeks. It turned out to be a medication problem, but when he couldn't sit, walk, or talk, I panicked. You see, when someone suffers an MS relapse, it's as if the nasty disease shouts, *"SURPRISE!"*

The events are scary because they shine a light on finality. How much time together do we have left? Will he remain weak, or will he bounce back? What will happen when I can't take care of him anymore?

I got good advice from the woman who counseled me at the ADRC. When I told her I felt defeated, she reminded me no one can assume all the duties which are required to help a patient like Ken. So I left feeling better, maybe even a little bit stronger. One can hope. I'll have to see what tomorrow brings.

IT'S GOOD TO DREAM

I 've always had a vision someday I would write a best seller from a desk which looks out to the ocean. The room would be large with an old oak desk facing the outdoor vista. Opened patio doors would let in the sound of crashing waves which would open my imagination, while the breeze keeps me cool. And of course, next to the desk there is a comfy overstuffed chair for my faithful writing pug pal Ernie to rest while I work.

One time I did some counseling to get over a "speed bump" in my life, and one of the techniques the therapist used was for me to go to a safe place in my mind and feel good about being there. My imaginary writing room does that for me now, especially on challenging days like yesterday.

In my writing room, I see my paintings surrounding me. They are hung on walls painted the palest shade of yellow. The flooring is a warm honey oak covered by one of my grandmother's hand-braided rugs. A cornflower blue sofa with geometric print ac-cent pillows provide a cozy seating area, while a ceiling fan keeps the room a pleasant temperature. On the opposite wall there is a fireplace for any cold, damp nights. The fire place opening is surrounded by beautiful, handmade Mexican tiles.

Bookcases flank each side of the fireplace which support my favorite books and photos of my friends and family.

Until the royalties come rolling in, I'll be satisfied to sit in my old, tattered chair with Ernie by my side. Ken sits across from me, and I look out to the quiet cemetery across the street. Our electric fireplace keeps us toasty on damp days. Our living room is as close to my dream as it can be right now.

Dreams are wonderful, but living in the present with what we have is even more important. So we do both . . . look to the future in our dreams and be thankful for what we have right now.

WAKING TO A SURPRISE

I'm sure I've mentioned my reaction to waking up to the sonic boom of Ken falling. This morning, I woke to his snoring. It wouldn't have been so unusual, but neither of us was in bed.

Often I wake up at two or three o'clock in the morning with pain. I have arthritis in my right hip, and if I lay on that side for too long, it will ache. So, I often drag myself out of bed, shuffle off to the bathroom, and take some ibuprofen to ease the pain and eventually go back to sleep.

Ordinarily, I go out to the living room and lay on the couch because it's softer than the bed and kinder to my sore hip. Of course, Ernie follows me and gets comfortable beside me. Then I turn on the television because by now, I'm wide awake and will need at least an hour before I'm sleepy enough to return to slumber.

So, now you understand why waking to Ken's snoring this morning was puzzling. I sat up, looked around the living room, and there he was fast asleep on the floor. As soon as I stirred, he woke up.

"What in the heck are you doing on the floor, dear?" I asked.

"I got up and all of a sudden, I got so weak, I just lowered myself to the floor and went to sleep."

"You're all right?"

"Yup." He said and struggled to stand. "What's for breakfast?"

I guess it's true—a way to a man's heart *is* through his stomach. "It's three o'clock in the morning. How about we go back to sleep and wake up at a more civilized hour. I'll make you French toast."

"Ah, you know how to bribe me."

"Hey, whatever works."

We laughed and cuddled to go back to sleep.

TAXING TIMES

I always put off filing taxes until the first week of April. So this April first I went onto the Turbo-Tax website, filled out the information required and happily learned I have a refund coming both from federal and state. Yeah!

The only problem is, the IRS won't accept my return because they cannot verify my identity. They will not give me an e-PIN number, and won't accept my AGI from last year. So, I fixed what I thought was wrong and tried again, only to have the damn thing bounce back yet again. I'm in an electronic looping nightmare. I have two choices, hopefully get an IRS rep on the phone to help me, or I can file by mail.

I wouldn't mind filing by mail, but I can't print the forms because my printer has run out of ink, which means before I can do anything I must go to the office supply store and buy new printer cartridges. Ouch. The cartridges are sixty dollars. Somedays things just don't go as planned. Besides trying to file taxes, I also have been going 'round and 'round with the mortgage company. They escrow my insurance premium in my monthly mortgage payment, but yet they didn't pay the bill — so the insurance company is taking withdraws from my bank account. So far, this hasn't been resolved, either.

Don't get me wrong — I love technology and shortcuts, but when things don't work the way they are supposed to work, I want to pull my hair out.

Oh, and by the way, this wasn't an April Fool's joke. It's the truth. Nothing but the truth.

LAUGHTER – WHO KNEW?

I love to laugh. From a giggle to a belly laugh, from a snicker to an all-out, tear rolling, uncontrollable breathtaking laugh—for me, laughter comes often and easy. I can make a joke out of most everything, and I truly believe it is one my best traits.

Yesterday, Dr. Oz—you know, Oprah's favorite doctor—talked about the benefits of having a good chuckle. So, like the researcher I am, I went out into Internet-land to see what I could find. I wanted my research to have the underpinnings of good scientific studies, so I turned to WebMD.

My Findings:

- We change physiologically when we laugh. We stretch muscles throughout our face and body, our pulse and blood pressure go up, and we breathe faster, sending more oxygen to our tissues. In fact, laughter has the same benefit of a mild workout.
- Combine laughter and movement and you boost your heart rate. Go out and walk, a laughing we will go!

- We burn calories when we laugh. — No Really. I kid you not. This is not a ploy to eat more chocolate. A researcher from Vanderbilt University claimed laughter appears to burn calories. Ten to fifteen minutes of laughter burns fifty calories.
- When your stress is high, your immune system decreases. So, if you're in a plague or a flu outbreak, laugh in its face! Take that, you nasty virus! The ability to use humor raises the level of infection-fighting antibodies in the body and boosts immune cells.
- Laughter lowers blood sugar levels. Hear that borderline diabetics? Raise your laughter, lower your sugar.
- Laughter dulls pain. I know this to be true from my own experience. When I broke my tibia in a sledding accident when I was fourteen years old, I cracked jokes and laughed through the whole experience. The doctor couldn't believe I wasn't screaming.

So, have I discovered the cure for what ails you? Not exactly.

So far, the lab boys and girls haven't proven beyond a shadow of a doubt the health benefits of laughing. Studies have been too small and not well-conducted according to a WebMD article. And because laughter is usually a social activity, scientists don't know if it's the laughter which actually improves health or whether improvement comes from being close with friends and family.

However, I'm definitely in the camp which maintains laughter undeniably improves your quality of life. Ken and I laugh all day long. To prove it, here's a conversation we had yesterday after watching Dr. Oz.

Me – "Do you believe it? Dr. Oz said laughing burns off more calories than sex."

Ken says with his dry wit. "Yeah, but he didn't say how many calories you would burn if you laughed during sex!"

What a guy! What a gift.

THE "I CAN'T" PRISON

My Dad turned eighty-nine on April 16. He's as proud of achieving this age as anyone turning twenty-one. And he's not alone. His best friend, Roy, is eighty-nine, too. In fact, the two of them are going to see who can make it to ninety first.

Roy and Dad have been friends since they were three years old. Both men are still full of hell. I can only imagine the trouble they got into as young boys and teenagers because they both are still mischief makers. So, what is the difference between them?

My Dad is in a nursing home, and Roy visits him.

Needless to say, in eighty-six years, Roy and my Dad have gone through thick and thin together. The difference is Roy still runs a business from his home, he travels, and constantly tries new things. He built a lightweight plane and flew it. He even learned how to ski at age seventy because he could do it for free at his "old" age.

The difference between them isn't health. Roy has had heart trouble and cancer, just like my Dad. Both men have had children die before them. Both men have had disappointments and joys in their long lives. So, what's the difference?

I think the difference is my father has always decided he wasn't good enough for more. He was reluctant to take a chance. He was cautious. He had a marvelous engineering mind, but he had no one in his life to encourage him. All he could see was a boy who had lost sight in one eye when he was injured in a "kick the can" accident. All he could see was a boy who only went to eighth grade. He married a woman who needed security, so he gave it to her by working at a steady job he hated for thirty years. I think hating to go to work every day brought on his bad health at a young age, so he had a legitimate excuse not to go back to the factory any longer. His arterial sclerosis and bad heart dictated long-term disability at age forty-eight.

I think we can all take a lesson from Roy and my Dad. Putting limits on yourself only allows you to proceed just so far. Fear of taking a chance has no benefit. Fear of making a mistake is a mistake. Success is in the failed attempts with the will not to quit.

If you fall in to the role of caretaker, you might feel trapped in the prison of *"I can't"* but you are wrong. The world doesn't have to stop spinning for you. Being home gave me the chance to write. Heck, I wrote seven novels and have another in the works. I also picked up a paint brush and explored painting with acrylics. I'm no Hemmingway or Monet, but these activities made me stretch and grow more than I ever imagined.

So the next time you want to say, "I can't," bite your tongue. Take a risk. Think outside the box. If you want to accomplish some-thing, it is possible. Perhaps not exactly the way you first imagined, but you can manifest new things into your life. Don't put yourself in the "I CAN'T prison." I don't think there's a worse place on earth.

PERSPECTIVE -- WHAT IS IT REALLY?

Early morning is my favorite time of the day. It's when our antique school clock keeps a steady beat, letting me know time marches on. It's when my dog sleeps beside me in my "woman and a dog chair" and Vinnie, our cat sits at my feet. It's a time when my thoughts are usually clear, and I can write without interruption. It's also a time when I often reflect on how lucky I am.

Some people might take a very different look at my life and see no happiness. They would see a woman who has been rolled over by corporate American enough times to have tread marks on her backside. They would focus on her unemployment for almost three years, except for an adjunct teaching job. They'd see a person whose credit rating plummeted and whose bank account has dried up. They would feel sorry for this woman whose husband suffers from MS leaving him lame with a loss of cognitive ability. Ten years ago he was a brilliant 3-D mechanical designer and now he can't do the math. They probably would see a person who has settled to live out her years in a small house with worn-out furniture.

But I have a different perspective from those people. I see the last several years as an opportunity to discover new abilities—like writing novels, creating handmade jewelry, and painting on canvas. Ken and I have ample time to enjoy each other playing a hot game of Scrabble on our back patio, while we sip an iced coffee and listen to the birds that live in the big trees on our lot. We have a chance to enjoy the antics of our furry kids.

I've learned perspective determines what kind of life you build. Ken and I have learned to lean in when life throws us a curve, and we run fast when we knocked the challenge out of the park. Everybody has a choice of striking out or hitting it over the fence. I think it all boils down to perspective.

161

WHEN TWO BRAINS ARE BETTER THAN ONE

When a person has a debilitating disease, he/she is always on the lookout for something to cure his/her curse or at least make a life a little bit better. Because we live in a "drug" culture, help often come in a pill, a syringe, or an infusion. This morning I saw a story about some research going on at Duke University. They interviewed a researcher who is exploring how a damaged brain and a healthy brain of another person can be networked to overcome the disability.

Sounds a little like science fiction, huh?

Well, they have had success with primates, getting the monkey to do things monkeys are not supposed to be able to do. But the research is preliminary. The power of the mind involves one hundred billion neurons and capturing their power is limitless. Just think of the implications this new approach could mean for MS and other brain injuries. If we can eliminate problems with the brain — and there is a very long list — wouldn't that be a miracle?

If this research offers a cure for stroke patients, wouldn't that be a blessing?

I don't think people should live forever, but I do think those patients who slip away a little piece at a time or lay in a nursing home because the treatments have been exhausted is inhumane. Generally, our culture doesn't condone assisted suicide, so people who are stricken with brain injuries or disease must wait for death to release them from their pain and disabilities. I believe such a policy is not fair to the patient or the family who cares for them. If brains can be networked with a small device and a better life can be achieved, I truly think we have advanced the entire human race.

Stories like this provide hope and possibility. Ken and I dream something like this will happen in our lifetime, and we'll be able to dance together again.

WHEN THE WORLD GETS TOO HEAVY

WHEN DISAPPOINTMENT RAINS DOWN

I often accept disappointment like a young child. Usually I pout and carry on like I'm the only person in the world who didn't get her way, and afterward I hate myself for behaving like a brat.

I think it's important to express anger in a controlled way. Just like every process, this is a learned activity for me. Caregiving presents frequent disappointments and frustrations, but underneath both is the fear of what might be down the road.

Ken is going through a stable period, but the unknown future scares the life out of me. People say I shouldn't borrow trouble, and they're right. I realize I shouldn't think about what MIGHT happen. But I'm being honest here—that's easier said than done.

When I've taken the appropriate amount of time to digest a disappointment, I will be my old self again. I'll wear a smile and when asked how I am, I'll say, "I'm fine." After all, most people expect that response, don't they?

THE ANNUAL TURKEY DINNER

The long Thanksgiving Holiday in America is over for another year. Only this time, we had to spend it alone.

Usually we join Ken's family for a big feast at his brother's home, but this year, Ken was just too fatigued to go. Thank goodness I've learned to always have a "Plan B."

Just in case such a situation might present itself, I had a substitute turkey dinner waiting in the wings. Along with the bird, I made his favorite scalloped corn, sweet potatoes, cranberries —the whole nine yards. It's great we both enjoy leftovers because we'll be eating turkey casseroles, stuffing and mashed potatoes, and of course we also eat sandwiches that rival the best deli. I'll use the carcass to make soup, and there's always a little bit of meat I freeze to enjoy turkey after I think I can't face another leftover.

Situations like this happen more and more frequently. We must live in the moment because everything depends upon Ken's health. We miss being with family members but so few people ever get a chance to experience a *Norman Rockwell* Thanksgiving.

That image we remember was a magazine cover for crying out loud. Having a happy holiday is a matter of perspective and living in the paradigm we're given. Our dinner for two Thanksgiving celebration turned out okay.

In another month Christmas will be here and the same scenario may repeat. Only then I'll be putting ham on the menu.

LIGHTING UP THE HOLIDAY

Today is December 1st – Let the Christmas festivities begin! Really? Merchants have had Christmas stuff on display for over two months now, which really irks me because I'm a purist. I think Halloween and Thanksgiving should be celebrated before the stores start hauling out the gold, red, and green blinking lights and other bobbles.

This year, though, I'm not feeling it.

To get in the spirit, I took a walk through a couple Christmas Tree Wonderlands at garden centers. As I wandered through the sea of lighted trees, I must say, it did the trick. I let the twinkling lights work their magic.

I remembered a time when I was a child, and my family piled into the Buick to "see the lights." Several neighborhoods were famous for putting up Christmas displays, so we appreciated the sights with "ooos" and "ahhhs" as we fogged up the car windows. The grand finale was always at a house at 6509 Williamsburg Way on the north side of the city.

Mr. George Wheary, a wealthy industrialist, delighted the entire city with an extravaganza of twenty-one thousand white lights in his yard. There were doves and angels "flying" in the large pine trees. The moon and constellations of the stars were there, too, but the centerpiece of the whole display was the 24-by-36 foot waterfall which had 2,000 feet of rope lights, creating the illusion of cascading water. This tasteful, beautiful scene of white lights lit up the cold winter nights. Everyone who made the effort to drive by the scene left awestruck. Fifty years ago, outdoor Christmas lights were an extravagance most people couldn't afford, so Mr. Wheary's lights imprinted memories which have lasted a lifetime.

This year the garden center lights helped me shake off my holiday funk, and I created my own winter light wonderland while Ken watched me from the window. I placed green garland with white lights on the railing of the wheelchair lamp with a wreath in the front. I used silver bows as accents. A big blue snowflake was wired to the wrought iron railing, and a white star projecting six different lighting patterns blinked brightly enough to land airplanes. The crowning beauty was the five-foot angel I fell in love with at Big Lots. After dark, I switched on the lights and gave myself a Christmas present.

When I came into the house, Ken had hot chocolate and cookies waiting for me, along with a big hug. "Sweetheart, it looks beautiful! It really seems like Christmas now."

He gave me the best gift of all.

WHEN THE FUNK SETS IN

Have you ever had a time in your life when procrastination took over? I'm in the midst of one of those times right now. It's December 11th and I still haven't put up my Christmas tree. I've hauled out other decorations and spread them around the house, but I just haven't been able to move myself to decorate the tree this year.

I told myself over the weekend, a cold, rainy day would be perfect for getting the tree up, but I watched football games instead. I'm sure this confession seems contrary because I've led everyone to believe I'm Mrs. Claus extraordinaire.

During our earlier travels, Ken and I always bought a Christmas ornament on our trips, so every year when we put the tree up, we fondly remembered our adventures together. I think his inability to help with the tree any more is why I'm dragging my feet. I'm also bummed because we won't be collecting any more ornaments.

I think my funk is more serious than just feeling lazy. I've been putting off everything. I've failed to go to the grocery store, so the cupboards have little to offer. I still haven't wrapped Christmas presents. Heck! I don't even know if I have a gift for everyone. Sending out Christmas cards is completely out of the question. Even making a simple, good, meal has been a chore lately, and I LOVE to cook. Worst yet, I haven't written too much of anything for weeks. I haven't had the energy to face my new novel. I've been a slug. I feel ashamed I'm dragging my feet, but all I want to do is play Facebook games.

I have nothing to be blue about. This year has been a good one for us. The wheelchair ramp and van has made it possible for us to get out. We've been blessed with very generous gifts of cash from a "Secret Santa" so we'd have presents under the tree.

I hate to face the answer to this. I must be depressed. After weeks of this behavior, I need help. Thank God, I was strong enough to pick up the phone and make an appointment with the doctor.

Caregiving is hard work and feeling down some of the time comes with it, but if you find you're in a rut like me, it's time to get help. It's not failure. There's no disgrace in seeking out help. I'm glad I did. A prescription of an antidepressant has helped me get back in gear in a couple of days.

Today I find myself decorating the house and receiving joy from all of the Christmas stuff we've collected over twenty years. Ken told me he really enjoys the decorations, especially the colored lights. His comment was just enough to ward off any other holiday funks.

WHEN IT'S TIME FOR A RESPITE

GETTING OUT OF DODGE

B eing a caretaker impacts a person in ways you never expect. As
you have read, Ken's Multiple Sclerosis can be scary and frustrating. I must continually remind myself what he does is the disease and not him, but sometimes I wish someone would release me
from this situation. I want to be a brat and stomp my foot claiming
"It's not fair!"

It's been four years since I've had a vacation, and that's way too
long. I need a change of scenery to recharge my battery, so I've
planned a four-day getaway to Florida to see my friend Kay. I'm not
getting away from Ken; I'm temporarily leaving my situation.

I've had to accept his illness is not my illness. I had to accept I
am worth having a life separate from his, even though I love him
more than anyone else in the world. My heart needs to stay
home, but my head realizes without a break I might snap. My
patience has waned, and I'm afraid I'll do or say something I will
regret. I also have to realize in order to continue to take care of
him, I have to take care of me first. If my "giving tank" is empty, I
will burn out and be of no use to him or myself.

Because Ken would rather stay home than go to a care center, the quest is more difficult. I need to find qualified people to provide care for him. I went to work with our coordinator who said she'd work with the home nurse to help me get this done.

It boils down to letting go. I have to trust the people who will care for Ken while I'm away. The "Life Alert" button he wears around his neck will help him stay safe for the hours he will be alone. The dinners I froze from leftovers of his favorite food will get him through the four days I'll be gone. I've done all I can to make this trip as easy for him as I can.

I only wish I was planning a trip with him as a healthy man. We loved traveling together and have taken many wonderful trips together. Timeshares in different parts of the country. A couple of cruises. Weekend getaways in quaint Bed & Breakfast places or swanky hotels. I am thankful for all of the good times we've share, but I'm also sad we'll probably never have a chance to explore the world together again.

AN HOUR OF REVELATION

Yesterday I had the pleasure of visiting with an old friend. We haven't been close through the years, but we've always had a presence in each other's life. We met when her son and my daughter were in nursery school together about forty years ago. Pam and I traveled a similar path through raising children, divorce, working, going to college later in life, belonging to the same church, etc. But we never grew close. That is changing now. Now a similar life experience has drawn us together again. We are both caretakers for someone we love. She for her mother. Me for Ken.

So every Thursday for the past few weeks, we've made a date with each other to do something together. We may meet for coffee or for lunch. Or she might just come over to our house and visit. Today she intends to show me the latest in the Mary Kay cosmetic line because she sells the stuff when she's not taking care of her Mom.

Somehow we never got around to Mary Kay. Instead we spent the sunny afternoon talking and laughing. During the course of our time together, she told me something which really surprised me.

She recalled a time when I had peach and apple trees growing in my backyard. At that time in my life I canned the fruit in Mason canning jars. She also remembered the jams and pies I made from the fruit trees which always gave me too much of a good thing and lots of work. She said she thought I did marvelous things. I never thought someone would see something like putting up preserves as marvelous.

I had grown up helping my mother can or freeze everything from green beans to strawberries every summer. Like little squirrels we prepared for the winter, preserving the fruits and vegetables my grandfather grew in his oversized garden. Mom and I needed to work in the summer to have enough to eat in the winter. My mother didn't work outside the home, and my father was an assembler in a muffler factory, so there wasn't any money to spare.

What is so amazing about this story is someone saw a simple process like canning as miraculous. There's a lesson to be learned here. What we take for granted in ourselves, others see as wonderful and special.

We all do special things. It's too bad it takes someone else to realize it.

FINDING PEACE

D id you ever have a day when you just wanted to growl at somebody? Yeah. You read correctly. I wanted to growl today. I'm
writing because I was afraid any word escaping from my mouth
might be toxic.

Ordinary when I feel like this, I just go out to my backyard and
drink a cup of coffee and let my flower garden simmer me down.
However, with my father's death, I received an inheritance which
allowed me to make several changes to our home as well as build a
new garage. Now the backyard is a pit because the city stalled our
garage building project, which also pushed back the landscaping
we want to do. Let's put it this way, no solace would be found in the
backyard this year.

I never want to take my crankiness out on Ken, so made sure
he was okay and got into the car and drove. I didn't have a destination, so I let the car take me where it wanted to go.

The car stopped at a garden center. I got out and pushed a cart
through the aisles and all of a sudden I felt better. As I got deeper
into the lot, I realized the perennials were discounted today, so
about a half dozen of them jumped into my cart.

As I stood in the checkout line, thirty or forty minutes later, I looked forward to planting my purchases in the flower garden that runs along the side of the new driveway. Walking through this beautiful place did the trick. I no longer felt crabby. I felt at ease and ready to get on with my weekly chores.

I guess it's true. Nature does calm the inner beast—even if "nature" is a garden center.

Respite can come in small packages.

DREAMS CAN BE RESPITES TOO

I t's Sunday morning. I look forward to this day every week. Why? Because when my favorite television program airs. Yes, I watch television. I am not ashamed to admit it. Other writing snobs brag they don't have time for the "lost wasteland," but television has brought me many hours of information and enjoyment. Besides, just because some people choose to not indulge in "the tube," it doesn't mean I have to be one of them.

Sunday is when CBS presents positive news. I see stories about the best of humanity—art, music, theatre, movies, new books and special events. Some stories even include the obscure—Bill Geist usually finds those. One of my favorites was about a retirement community in Florida where the residents get around in custom-designed golf carts which look like a Rolls Royces, Ferraris, Mustangs or any other dream car. The community also had everything retirees need -- a grocery store, barbershops, a bank, restaurants, etc. The only thing missing was a hospital.

When I saw that piece, I wanted to move the next day. I dreamed of ordering my own '56 Thunderbird golf cart complete with pink, fuzzy dice hanging from the rear-view mirror and "dragging" down the main street with another resident in his '57 Chevy!

This one weekly program presents stories I would not see anywhere else. Today they did a piece on a Japanese woman artist who has risen to fame by painting polka-dots. She suffered a horrific childhood and paints pictures using polka-dots because this simple dot helped her maintain her sanity. Now, she is world renown and has been hired by a famous designer for a new line. Isn't it amazing what the human spirit can do?

Charles Osgood is a perfect host of this program. He's a an older man who wears a bow-tie and stands alone to present the stories in his smooth, single-malt voice. On top of his suave appeal, he is extremely talented on the piano. I feel cheated when someone else fills in for him.

When I started watching this program over twenty years ago, I dreamed when I made it BIG, I would watch a piece on Sunday Morning and have the means to go and see the ballet, concert or play in person. I would pick up the phone and have my personal secretary make the arrangements for me to fly to the destination, see the production, stay in a 5-star hotel, and then fly home the next day.

So far, I'm still working on that. Dreams can be a respite too.

QUEEN FOR A DAY

Once a year the Aging and Disability Resource Center in our area invites caregivers to a special luncheon. The theme this year was a "Virtual Cruise." Having enjoyed at least ten cruises in my lifetime, I wondered how they would carry this off.

The theme was set at the front door when we all were met with an "Aloha" greeting, while a colorful silk lei was placed around our necks. Ken and the other patients would spend the day being cared for by professionals in a separate room.

Caregivers were ushered down a long hallway where Hawaiian music wafted through a grand ballroom. Large round tables covered in white linen each had a silk star lily centerpiece. We were invited to sip a drink from tall, tropical glasses with paper umbrellas. The only thing missing in the fruity drinks was the rum.

From ten o'clock until two o'clock approximately fifty caregivers enjoyed an afternoon of relaxation and laughing. We were encouraged to learn about some of the services available to us when we need extra help. The organizers had a clever way to get us to visit all of the vendors by giving us a "passport" which needed to be stamped by each vendor as we completed our "worldwide tour." The passports were then collected for door prize drawings at the end of the day.

I didn't win a thing, but I did have a nice day out of the house. Our group enjoyed entertainment including teenage dancers, a ventriloquist, and a massage therapist, who gave five-minute chair massages to anyone who wanted one. When it was my turn, I was flabbergasted he found such sore, tight muscles on both sides of my shoulders. I guess I really needed a "cruise."

During the ride home, Ken said he had a good time. Two people from his "Harmony Club" were there. But I never worry about Ken in a social setting; he's so congenial he can talk with anyone.

If you're a caregiver, I hope you have such support in your community. I've found caring and helpful people in our local Aging and Disability Center. It took me too long to pick up the phone and call them. What a dope.

Be smarter than me. Don't wait until you want to pull your hair out to call your local agency. Besides being caring and empathetic, the people there are connected to services which will help. They also help to keep things in perspective. They understand your anger, frustration, and the need for answers. Best of all these people know how to maneuver through the obstacles and restrictions all caretakers face.

BACK TO MECCA AGAIN

I 'm spending a week in Florida in the middle of a Wisconsin winter. It's thirty degrees at home, but today in Orlando it's in the eighties, and I'm enjoying paradise beside a large pool which is surrounded by three-story palms and tropical flowers.

It's quiet in the early morning. With pen in hand, I begin to write. I've had a long dry spell, and I'm hoping to get started again. I'm sitting under a colorful umbrella, which is stuck in the middle of a metal table. Tropical music plays in the background. It's a contrived Caribbean atmosphere, but the mood has conjured up memories I'd long forgotten.

I met Robin and Jane over twenty years ago during a cruise. It wasn't long before the three of us became good friends. They were travel agents and when they wanted a companion on a FAM trip, they'd call me. At the time, I called these excursions "mental health" trips because I could escape the bitterness of my nasty divorce. Together we experienced many of the islands which lay in the amazing aqua waters of the Gulf of Mexico and the Caribbean Sea.

Then I ran away from my life for a week, and I suppose someone could see this trip as the same thing. I'm recharging my emotional batteries in the sunshine. Like my cruises with Jane and Robin, this trip will help me change my perspective.

I hear different languages surrounding me, and children saying "Marco Polo" again and again. I watch little girls and boys frolic with their parents, and I wonder where life will take them. Childhood goes so fast. Before a person can take a breath, gray hair and creaky joints replace the nimbleness of our younger years. I remember being six and wanting to be seven. Sixteen wanting to be twenty-one. Like most young people, I rushed through my youth wishing to get to adulthood on the fast track. Youth really is wasted on the young, isn't it? At this stage I wish I could take my lifetime of knowledge and go back and live life all over again.

The breeze has become a brisk wind, so I move to the chaise I claimed with a towel. I had hoped the sun would show up, but fast moving clouds have prohibited the orb from making an appearance today. I spy a beautiful yellow flower and decide to take a photo of it, so when I return home, I can paint it.

A man sitting nearby strikes up a conversation. "Do you know what kind of flower that is?"

I look up and smiled. "No. I just think it's pretty, and I want to take it home with me."

"Where's home?"

"Wisconsin. Where are you from?"

"Michigan. A suburb of Detroit. I'm Paul, by the way." He smiles.

And so it goes. We engaged in small talk for the next few minutes.

He's very attractive with just enough gray in his hair to realize he's no kid. His eyes are shaded by expensive sunglasses, and his pressed trousers and starched business shirt shouts he's well off. He wore no jewelry except for a Rolex on his wrist. He tells me he's a commercial banker. I tell him I had been a financial advisor for about six years. In the next breath I tell him I'm my husband's caregiver. Why did I say that? Before my eyes he tenses up and adjusts his position in the chair. Our easy conversation turns uncomfortable in a moment. Which makes me wonder why he initiated this conversation in the first place. Did he see me as a woman who might be interesting? Then in a few words I confessed my world is small.

I noticed he had a workbook on the table with a pen resting on top of it. "Looks like you have some homework."

He cleared his throat. "Yeah. I'm supposed to fill this booklet before I go to a ten o'clock meeting."

"Then I'll let you get to it. It was nice talking with you, Paul."

"Likewise." He smiled and turned his back to me.

The encounter was brief. I hate to admit I liked his attention. I guess I'm not too old to desire a little attention from a handsome man. It's been a long time since I experienced such a thing. Ken used to always notice me, but during the past few years I've become a fixture. He always used to tell me I looked nice; now such a comment is a rarity.

I realize I must take care of me in order to care for Ken, but it's easier just to sit in a chair and let the world go by. I vow when I get home I'll make an effort to structure my day to include some exercise, but again, I won't tell anyone about my intentions because then I'd have to stick to it. As Ken's needs increase, I push myself into the background to get through the long days.

Last night I ate an expensive meal at the "tapa" tavern which is in the lobby of the hotel. If I made a habit of eating small portions like that all of the time, I wouldn't be lamenting about my out-of-shape body. Easier said than done.

I'm at this hotel with my good friend Kay for two nights during my week's stay with her. She thought the tropical atmosphere would be a good substitute for a place in the Caribbean. We joke someday we'll bar tend in colorful island dresses making drinks for patrons on a beach somewhere.

We'll leave the hotel tomorrow at noon, and then the next day I'll leave for home. I'm ready to go, and Ken is ready for me to come home. He tells me my pug dog Ernie has been keeping vigil in the front window for me to return, and Vinnie our cat has given up his nighttime treats.

I'm thankful for this week to do nothing important. I've slept late. Visited with my friend. Laughed at her cats and even snooped the local flea market. I've purchased presents for all my loved ones at home and even splurged on a wild tropical blouse for myself. Kay has waited on me like I'm royalty. This trip is just what I needed.

As I pack my suitcase, I'm extraordinarily quiet. I guess I'm gearing up for what my day-to-day life holds. Three hours on a plane isn't long enough to make a complete transformation, but it's what I have. As soon as I open the door at home, I'll be once again thinking for two people, cleaning up messes, and finding solace in the quieter moments life provides. But it's okay. I've chosen this life because I love Ken. It's as simple as that.

A DIFFERENT KIND OF RESPITE

When most people think of the word respite, they envision a happy time. My most recent respite is anything but happy.

About a month ago, Ken got very sick. He developed a Urinary Tract Infection—UTI for those medical personnel out there. We were both surprised. He exhibited no symptoms except for extreme fatigue and the inability to speak intelligibly. When he hallucinated in the ER, seeing things that weren't in the room, I realized how sick he really had become.

What this meant was a four-day stay in the hospital with intravenous antibiotics followed by a month of rehab in a nursing home. The time we had been dreading for over ten years has finally surfaced. We will be separated for an extended time.

The infection took its toll on Ken but I think it also affected his MS. His right leg is no longer functioning, and he must rest frequently to get through the day. He does his best with physical therapy; in fact his therapist told me yesterday (after him being away from home for three weeks) that Ken walked forty feet. That's more walking than he's done in years. So we both are hopeful he will be able to come home soon. The problem right now is his behavior is not consistent from day to day.

The last three weeks have allowed me to get some much needed rest. I didn't realize how much Ken's care takes out of me. His incontinence alone keeps me very busy cleaning him up and washing the clothes.

We're both hoping he'll be coming home soon, but no hard-set plans are in place as of this writing. The social worker and the nurse at the rehab center are working to come up with a plan which will work for both of us.

Somedays I fear this "respite" will go on forever.

EPILOGUE

As the journey with Multiple Sclerosis goes forward, I've discovered the hardest part of this disease is not knowing what will happen from day to day. The doctors have labeled Ken's case as "progressive MS." He's had a steady decline over the past ten years, but he's also had periods when he's faltered one day and felt fine the next.

We find it harder and harder to schedule outings. We've had to educate our friends and family we can only make tentative or spur-of-the-moment plans because we never know if Ken will be strong enough to make the trip. If a heavy load of fatigue falls on Ken, we call, negate the plans, and stay home. We can cry in our beer, or we can create a "Plan B". We've also learned keeping a positive attitude is not easy, but we do our best.

The best part of this experience is feeling the love from our friends and family. Few have deserted us. They Our show their concern with their pocketbooks and visits. They wrap their arms around us with unconditional love. We'll never live a "normal" life – whatever that is. Instead we'll live the best life possible with the gifts we are given.

That's good enough for us.

www.ingramcontent.com/pod-product-compliance
Lightning Source LLC
Chambersburg PA
CBHW071424170526
45165CB00001B/387

* 9 7 8 1 5 4 8 3 5 4 1 2 1 *